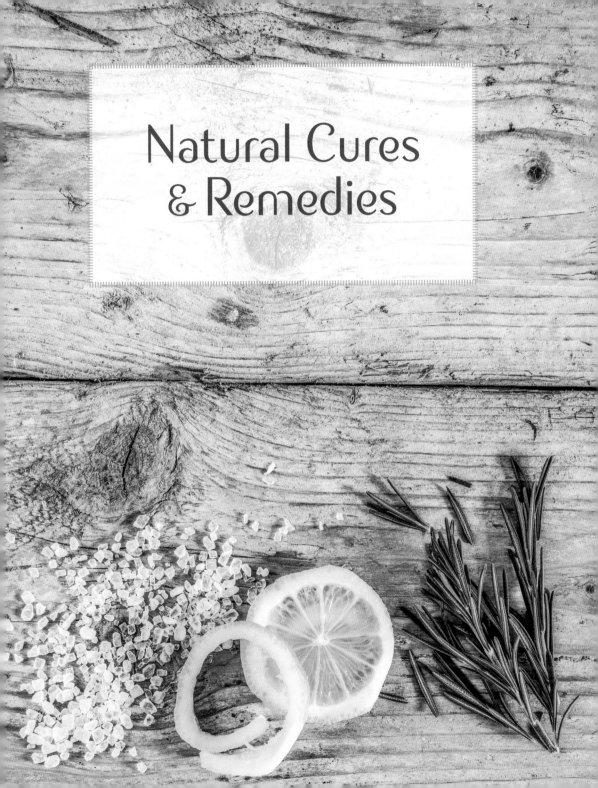

Natural Cures & Remedies

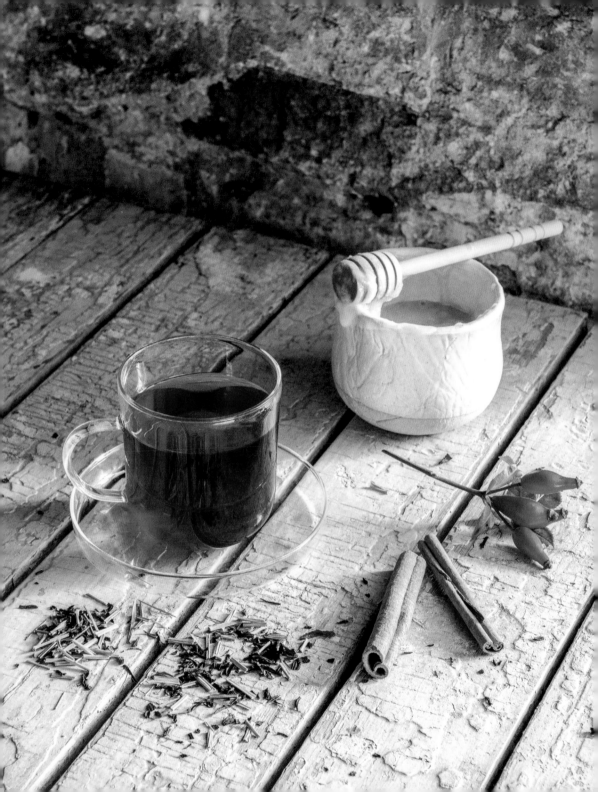

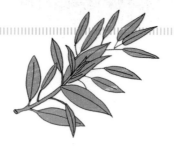

Natural Cures & Remedies

Kitchen cupboard recipes and solutions for your health and home

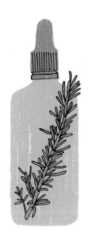

CICO BOOKS

LONDON NEW YORK

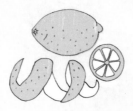

Published in 2021 by CICO Books
An imprint of Ryland Peters & Small Ltd
20–21 Jockey's Fields   341 E 116th St
London WC1R 4BW   New York, NY 10029

www.rylandpeters.com

10 9 8 7 6 5 4 3 2 1

A CIP catalog record for this book is available from the Library of Congress and the British Library.

ISBN: 978-1-80065-010-7

Printed in China

Illustrator: Rosie Lewis
Senior editor: Carmel Edmonds
Commissioning editor: Kristine Pidkameny
Senior designer: Emily Breen
Art director: Sally Powell
Head of production: Patricia Harrington
Publishing manager: Penny Craig
Publisher: Cindy Richards

Please note that if you are concerned about your health, you are advised to consult a doctor or physician. The information in this book should not be treated as a substitute for medical advice.

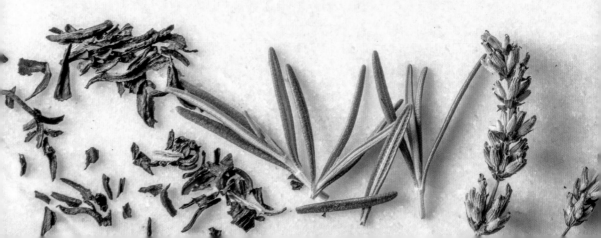

contents

introduction 6
useful herbs and spices 8

chapter 1
relieving aches, pains, and injuries 18

chapter 2
maintaining good health 38

chapter 3
enhancing mental well-being 62

chapter 4
beauty solutions 88

chapter 5
a healthy home and garden 118

resources 140
index 141
credits 143

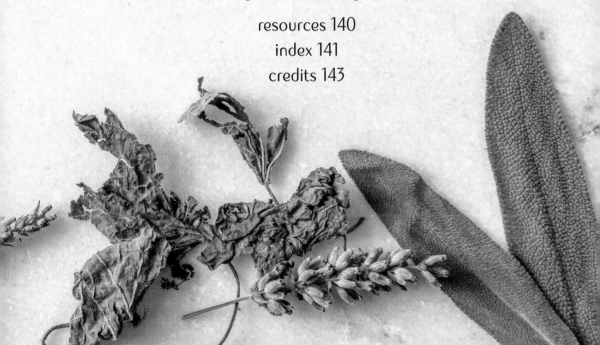

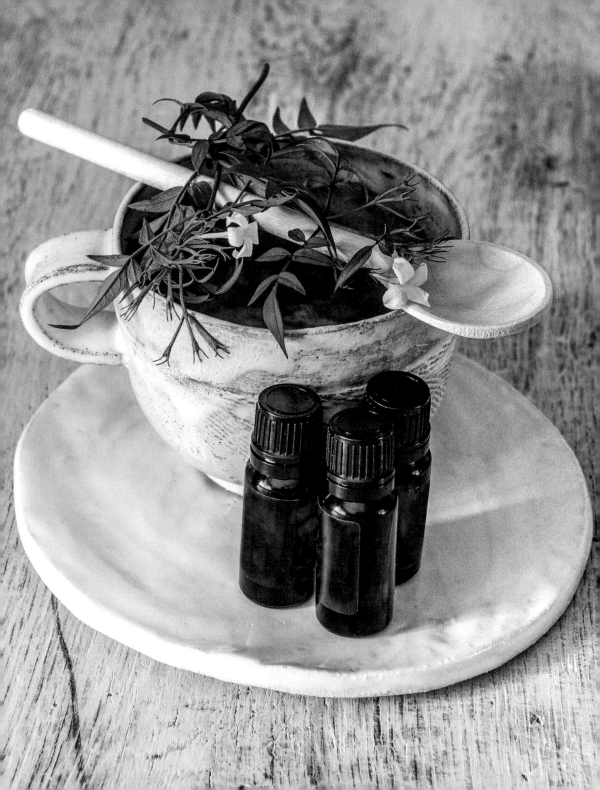

introduction

When our grandmothers and elders tended cuts, bruises, colds, fevers, and other illnesses their families suffered, they didn't have a corner drugstore. Instead, these wise women relied on simple wisdom, common sense, and pantries well stocked with herbal remedies. These preparations were made from plants that grew in the kitchen garden or from wild weeds gathered in the fields and woods surrounding their homes.

While we live in a modern world of cutting-edge clinics and advanced medicine, there is still much you can do using the natural remedies right from your pantry and kitchen garden, just like those who came before us. The roses blooming by your front gate contain more vitamins than the expensive bottle of chemicals on your bathroom shelf. Your spice rack is your closest pharmacy. Your home-brewed honey vinegar is a powerful tonic your family will love.

Not only will you save money with these homemade remedies but also, more importantly, you will begin to learn what works for you as you bring much comfort to yourself and your loved ones. So many of us are overwhelmed due to fragmented lifestyles requiring long hours at work, zillions of emails and text messages, social media, and all the other demands that don't stop flooding in. But cures made from natural ingredients encourage a connection to the earth and the cycles of nature, which helps maintain balance and harmony, and allows you to stay centered, grounded, and healthy.

As well as healing maladies, we can also care for our appearance in an all-natural way. Self-care involves, in great part, living in harmony with the seasons and the natural world. Using a lot of chemicals in your personal care products goes against this, so take stock of what your soaps, shampoos, and cleansers contain, and consider making your own, so that every ingredient is under your control.

We can look after our home, too. We all want to live somewhere that makes us feel happy and safe. The chemicals in our usual cleaning products introduce toxins into our lives. Who likes the smell of raw bleach, over-perfumed detergent, and scary oven cleaners? They strip away the natural and are simply too harsh. There are so many alternatives that are inexpensive and will make your home—and anyone who walks through the door—healthier and happier.

useful herbs and spices

This is a quick go-to guide to many common herbs, spices, and other foods and their medicinal uses.

HERBS

sage

When drunk as a tea or eaten, sage helps ease flatulence and bloating. It also helps to stop milk when a mother is weaning a baby, but should not be used if you think you may be pregnant other than as incense. It helps calm nervousness and anxiety, and boosts liver function. When applied externally to the skin, diluted sage essential oil (diluted in a carrier oil—see page 12) or fresh leaves can help heal insect bites, red skin, and soothe inflamed gums (due to teething, wisdom teeth, or toothache, for example) until you can get to a dentist.

oregano

When eaten, oregano can act as a stimulant to treat low energy or mild depression. Drunk as a tea, it can help tension headaches and bring on menstruation. It should never be used in pregnancy, or if you think you may be pregnant.

lavender

Lavender is used to treat unexplained muscle spasms such as eye twitches—you can rub a drop of the oil or the fresh or dried flower around the eye (being careful not to get any in the eye), or make a spray with a gentle oil such as almond and dried lavender, and spray over the face (with eyes closed), then massage in gently. Warm lavender baths help circulation, especially if you have cold hands and feet. A lavender compress can help lower fever. A lavender wash will help most skin issues, from oily skin and acne to insect bites, inflammations, and dermatitis.

marjoram

Marjoram tea eases bronchial coughs and can also help with tension headaches and anxiety. Drinking the tea and/or massaging some marjoram essential oil (diluted in a carrier oil—see page 12) into the lower stomach area can ease menstrual pain. Gently massaging the outer ear and the back of the ear with dilute marjoram oil can help cure ear infections. Marjoram essential oil should not be used during pregnancy, although using small amounts of the herb in cooking is generally considered safe.

peppermint

Its antispasmodic effects soothe the stomach after a big meal (drinking peppermint tea or eating a peppermint sweet, for example), or when experiencing morning sickness, gas, or colic. It is used, in conjunction with Western medicine, to treat irritable bowel syndrome.

rosemary

A rosemary-and-oil rub is said to help slow down hair loss by boosting the circulation; it also tones the scalp to avoid dandruff (wash your hair, massage in the rosemary and oil, leave for a few minutes, then wash again). Rosemary contains lots of iron and vitamin C, making it a great tea for the cold months of the year. While it is fine to eat rosemary-flavored foods during pregnancy, you shouldn't eat whole spoonfuls or use the essential oil at that time.

wild garlic

A cut garlic bulb applied to ringworm wounds or other skin infections can help heal them; eating garlic is said to lower cholesterol. It also stimulates the immune system, so is used in the treatment of colds and flu.

basil

Rubbed on the skin, crushed leaves or basil essential oil (diluted in a carrier oil—see page 12) can alleviate stress-induced skin issues, such as contact dermatitis. When taken in food, it encourages proper digestion and helps ease stomach cramps. Drinking basil tea when exhausted promotes relaxation and sleep—however, the taste can be a bit strong for most people. Basil should not be used when pregnant.

vervain

The leaves and root can be used in a tea (useful to increase breast milk and to stop diarrhea; it also has a general calming effect) and the flowers for edible decoration. Use crushed fresh leaves in a cool poultice to stop headaches. The Native Americans used to collect the seeds after flowering, roast them, and then grind them into flour used to make little bread-like rolls eaten before rituals.

feverfew

When drunk as a tea, feverfew can aid relief from migraine headaches; it also helps bring on a proper period when you are just spotting. The flowers can cause vomiting. Feverfew grows plentifully in hedgerows.

patchouli

Used to cover up other smells due to its pungent nature. The essential oil, diluted in a carrier oil (see page 12) and rubbed on the skin, can ease dry, chapped skin, acne, and prominent varicose veins.

bergamot

Bergamot is antiseptic; the tea, drunk with a dollop of honey, is used to treat colds, including low fevers and sore throats. It can also relieve flatulence.

citronella

Citronella is commonly used as an insect repellant—by placing the plant near open windows or outside on tables, burning citronella candles, or applying to the skin (cooled citronella tea or citronella essential oil diluted in spring water are common remedies). It can also help relieve excess sweating.

bay

Dried leaves and bay oil are used in cooking and have a mild stimulant effect. Bay leaves are antifungal and an extract of bay—3½ oz (100 g) of the herb to around 13½ fl oz (just under half a liter) of alcohol—can be used to treat athlete's foot and similar problems.

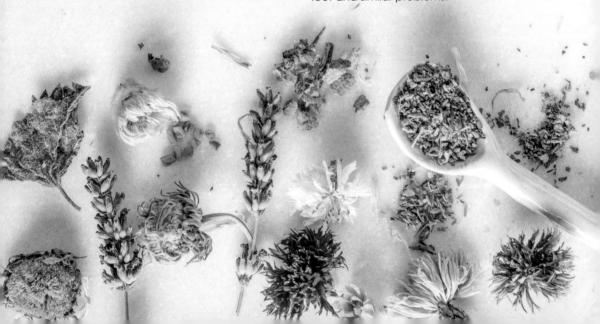

lemongrass

Lemongrass tea is drunk after an illness to boost the glandular, immune, and digestive systems. It also gives a general energy boost, relieves nervousness, and helps with jet lag. The crushed grass, or essential oil diluted in a carrier oil (see page 12), can be applied directly to the skin to relieve muscle spasms such as eye and mouth twitches, or leg cramps after exercise. Applied the same way to skin, it is also used to treat ringworm, other parasites such as lice, and athlete's foot.

dill

Dill aids digestion—add some dill seeds to a heavy dish or serve dill leaf tea after a big meal. It is great for relieving colic and the associated stomach upset, even in small children (see the gripe water recipe on page 27). Chew dill seeds to clear your breath after eating garlic, or just to freshen your breath. Dill rubbed on the skin promotes healing.

hawthorn

Hawthorn berry tea is drunk to improve circulation, especially in the hands and feet, and to lower blood pressure. The tea or syrup is also used in the treatment of insomnia and as a memory aid for older people or those who are stressed.

jasmine

Dab some cooled jasmine tea on red or burning eyes to ease them. A strong infusion, gargled, can be used to treat mouth ulcers. Jasmine is a great tonic for the skin—use on red or warm skin after sun and wind burn, or bathe in jasmine flowers or with a few drops of jasmine essential oil to treat dry and stressed skin (great for contact dermatitis). It can also be used to treat mild depression.

chamomile

Chamomile tea is used as a mild sedative, to cure insomnia, and to ease stomach cramps and aches, especially menstrual cramps. A cool tea or mild infusion given in a bottle or cup to teething babies will lessen discomfort. Great as an anti-inflammatory and to ease rheumatic pains, it can be applied as an ointment (see opposite) or by rubbing crushed flowers directly onto the skin. A salve applied externally will ease hemorrhoids and sunburn. Chamomile tea can also be used as a tonic for other plants.

chives

Chives may reduce blood pressure, help regulate blood sugar levels, and promote relaxation. Are you trying to stop smoking? Whenever you feel the need for a cigarette, chew some chives instead.

eucalyptus

This is great to help breathing when you have a cold or bronchial issues—boil some leaves and inhale the steam or add a few drops of eucalyptus essential oil to your bath. Make an ointment to have on hand for pulled muscles and sprains (see opposite). Undiluted essential oil, dabbed on abscesses and warts, will help them recede.

fennel

A few drops of fennel essential oil added to warm water as a drink can help with gas and heartburn, and will increase menstruation and urine flow as well as increase breast milk, but should not be used during pregnancy. Fennel syrup can ease a chronic cough. Gargle with cooled fennel tea to treat gingivitis and sore throats.

red clover

This is used to treat breathing and skin problems, as well as PMS. and is gentle enough to be used on children's skin. The tea can be drunk or, when cooled, applied to the skin, or the essential oil diluted in almond or rosehip oil, then applied.

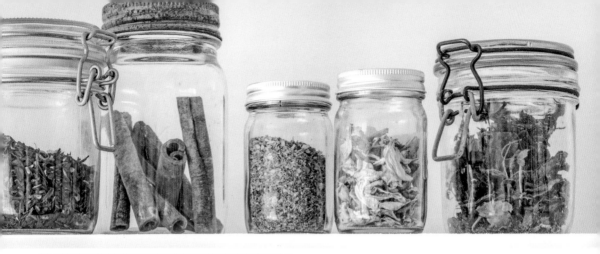

making an ointment

Ointments allow you to keep herbs for longer and gain their benefits within a salve or balm. To make an ointment, heat a pure, plain fat such as lard or petroleum jelly in a bainmarie (a bowl placed in hot water). When the fat begins to melt into liquid, stir in your essential oils or crushed fresh herbs—the amount depends purely on personal preference—and keep this semi-fluid for an hour or so, stirring often before pouring it into small jars or tins. It's best to use sterilized jars (see page 17), or at least wash them in a hot dishwasher first. Let the mixture cool and solidify before putting on lids; if you are using glass or other see-through containers, store them in a dark place. The ointment will last for around nine months. However, if you use inferior fat the ointment can go stale—you will know by the smell.

catnip

Catnip is great for repelling mosquitoes! Some cats act as if "high" on it. The plant can act as a stimulant or sedative for humans, so eat a little and test its effects first! Catnip also stimulates sweating and thus can help break a fever. A weak catnip infusion massaged into the scalp will reduce dandruff, and dabbed on swollen and puffy eyes will ease them. A strong catnip infusion can be used as a flea-repellent bath for animals or as an anti-flea shampoo for carpets.

pennyroyal

It can be taken as a tea to stimulate contractions when labor is slow starting. It should not be used in pregnancy until labor has begun, or if you think you may be pregnant.

wormwood

A few drops of wormwood essential oil in warm water can be drunk as a tonic and to reduce fever. It can also be used to treat worms in humans and animals. The leaves can be made into a tea, which eases pain and has traditionally been used to treat labor pain. The essential oil, diluted, is applied to soothe insect and snake bites and draw out the poison. Only use it in a very diluted form, as pure wormwood can be poisonous. The liquor absinthe is made from wormwood.

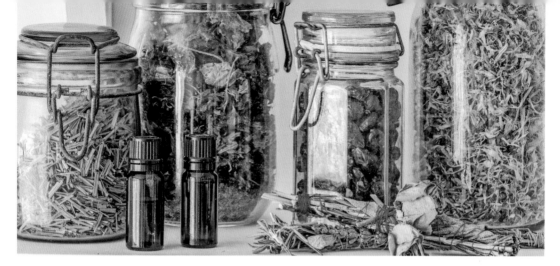

thyme

Drinking thyme tea or inhaling the steam from an infusion can ease coughs and tonsillitis. Thyme is antiseptic and antifungal, and gargling can help treat gingivitis and other gum diseases (gargle with strong cooled thyme tea, or with a few drops of the essential oil added to warm water). Make a strong infusion and massage into the scalp to treat a dry, itchy scalp and dandruff. While it is fine to eat thyme-flavored foods during pregnancy, you shouldn't eat whole spoonfuls or use the essential oil.

valerian

This is a great aid for any sleep issues, from general insomnia to stress-induced sleeplessness or noise issues. Strong valerian tea (made with the root) is given after a stressful event to ease the mind and body, and normal strength valerian tea can be drunk to ease PMS and menopausal symptoms.

buckthorn

Boiled with honey, buckthorn eases constipation and acts as a diuretic. Buckthorn tea is used to treat gallstones, in conjunction with Western medicine. It can be used as a purgative for animals, such as when a dog has eaten chocolate and needs to regurgitate it. Do not use it if pregnant or breastfeeding.

carrier oils

It is often easier to get hold of an essential oil than a fresh plant, so the uses of the herbs in this section often make mention of essential oils, which should be diluted in a carrier oil (sometimes called a base oil). Almond or rosehip oil are good options, but go with whichever oil you prefer—for example, you might like grapefruit, jojoba, or olive oil.

lemon balm

With antibacterial and antiviral properties, lemon balm can be applied to fresh insect bites to lessen itching and swelling. It is used in the treatment of cold sores and the herpes simplex virus—crush a leaf and apply directly, or use a strong cooled lemon balm tea. The tea also makes a refreshing drink to treat depression and anxiety. It's very easy to grow!

SPICES

nutmeg
Nutmeg used in foods will stimulate the appetite, especially after an illness, as it can help prevent nausea; will also help prevent flatulence by moving food along the intestinal tract. Used to treat minor morning sickness, nutmeg essential oil or a strong nutmeg infusion can also ease toothache and skin complaints, such as dermatitis and eczema.

cumin
Cumin prevents flatulence and bloating; it can be taken as a tea or, more commonly, simply chewed slowly.

allspice
This has antiseptic and slight anesthetic properties, and is used to help chest infections (usually eaten with food) and ligament and muscle pain (applied to the skin as a rub by adding the herb to a carrier oil—see opposite). Allspice encourages digestion and, because of this, is often an ingredient in after-dinner pastries and heavy Germanic winter breads. The berries are lovely in mulled wine and a tea or infusion brewed from the leaves is sometimes used to disguise the bitter taste of other medicinal herbs. The essential oil is used to treat stress and mild depression.

cardamom
This can be used to flavor coffee, and will lessen the effect of caffeine therein. It helps with PMS (when drunk as a weak tea) and, as a gargle, excess mucus in the mouth (such as after digesting dairy products or when suffering from a mild inflammation of the mouth). In larger amounts, it can have a laxative effect.

black pepper
This stimulates the taste buds and aids digestion, so is great to use when encouraging someone to eat, such as after an illness.

caraway seed
A tea can be drunk to ease stomach discomfort, especially to help heartburn and nausea, or as a gargle to help throat ailments, especially laryngitis. In some Asian countries, gently roasted caraway seeds are served after celebratory meals to aid digestion; it is also said to increase milk production in breastfeeding mothers.

star anise
This is used in tonics, and as a tea to ease coughs and colds and to clear the lungs; in ancient Egypt, the seeds were smoked for this purpose. Star anise essential oil (difficult to find) is a great antiseptic. Avoid the oil during pregnancy.

chili
This can ease pain, especially backache, and reduces itching. Usually the seeds are added to a cream or oil and applied to the skin, but chili is also effective when eaten in food.

cinnamon
Cinnamon is an astringent, a stimulant, and an antiseptic; sipping some warm water with a cinnamon stick swirled in it can help stop vomiting. The essential oil is famed for its antibacterial and antifungal properties, but also has other uses; a few drops mixed with some banana mash can help relieve flatulence and diarrhea. There is some evidence that eating a teaspoon of ground cinnamon a day can help with high cholesterol and reduce blood-sugar levels, but more research is needed. While it is fine to eat cinnamon-flavored foods during pregnancy, you shouldn't eat whole spoonfuls or use the essential oil at that time.

red peppercorn
When ingested, red peppercorn will ease constipation and is said to lower fever. Roughly ground and mixed with a carrier oil (see opposite), it can be rubbed on arms and legs to increase circulation.

clove

Chewing cloves, or drinking them in tea, can help with digestive issues, especially bloating and cramping. It can also help kill internal parasites, such as worms, and ease allergy and hay fever symptoms as it has mild antihistamine properties. If you have toothache, bite down on a clove to ease the pain until you can get treatment from a dentist.

mustard

Rubbing whole mustard seeds onto the skin can stimulate circulation and relieve muscle pain.

ginger

When eaten or drunk as a tea, it will stimulate the senses and prevent gas. Candied ginger is great for preventing and curing morning sickness and sea sickness. Juiced ginger is drunk to help with hangovers and diarrhea.

ADAPTOGENS

Adaptogens are herbs, superfoods, and other substances that have nonspecific actions on the body, meaning they support all the major systems as well as regulatory functions. They don't harm or cause additional stress to the body. Instead, they help the body adapt to many and varied environmental and physiological stresses, and they should be included in our diets to enhance and protect our immune and hormonal systems.

mucuna pruriens

Mucuna pruriens (also known as kapikachhu) is a legume that contains L-dopa, which is an amino acid found in the body that transforms into dopamine in the brain. Dopamine is a neurotransmitter that allows the dynamic functioning of the brain. Higher levels of dopamine can help with sleep, brain function, and an expanded sense of well-being. Mucuna pruriens is known for its ability to lift moods and enhance sexual function. You can use it in a sleep or energy tonic and it will work naturally for what your body needs most.

amalaki

Amalaki (or amla for short) tastes and smells amazing, and it's the ultimate beauty food. Amla nourishes the blood, detoxes and restores health to the liver, is rich in vitamin C, and is known as the immortality fruit. It can be purchased as both a herb and a powder, but the powder is best for tonics.

astragalus

Astragalus is an Ayurvedic root (bought as a powder) that is used to balance hormones, specifically cortisol levels. You'll find many popular herbal formulas contain astragalus nowadays because of the rise in people's stress levels. Astragalus helps balance those suffering from chronic fatigue, immune disorders, kidney disease, and high blood pressure.

pearl powder

Pearl powder, often used in Chinese medicine, is simply crushed pearls. Taking this adaptogen internally can boost collagen production and increase cellular turnover. Pearls are rich in calcium, which strengthens hair, teeth, and nails. Pearl powder for use in recipes should be labeled as food grade, but it sometimes isn't. However, you can use most pearl powder internally the same as externally, provided that it is pure and there is no filler in the powder (which would be listed under the ingredients).

ashwagandha

Ashwagandha is an adaptogenic herb that has been used for centuries to enhance youthfulness and reproductive function and nourish supple skin, lustrous shiny hair, and the internal organs for an all-over body glow. Ashwagandha is also known for its plethora of important minerals, including magnesium, which is a crucial mineral in the body that can help to soothe anxiety, alleviate depression, improve sleep, and has a calming effect on the body's physiological and nervous systems. Among many other great qualities, ashwagandha increases nitric oxide in the body, which is why it's known for its aphrodisiac qualities. The incredible thing about adaptogens is their multifunctional qualities. Not only does ashwagandha soothe the nervous system but it deeply energizes the body (although it's not a stimulant), balances hormones, and supports healthy adrenals.

moringa

Moringa is one of those miracle herbs that can be used for many ailments (like most adaptogens). Moringa slows the effects of aging, balances hormones, improves digestion, is rich in micronutrients, balances blood sugar levels, and is rich in protein. Moringa can be used in smoothies as well as face masks (see page 91) because it's packed with free-radical fighting antioxidants.

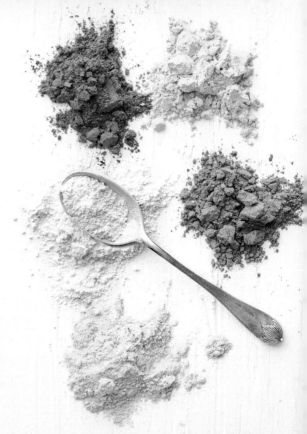

schizandra berry

Schizandra berry is a beauty adaptogen that focuses on the adrenals, liver, skin, and hormones. This beautifully tart berry increases libido, improves mental function, reduces inflammation, cleanses the liver, aids stomach-related imbalances, and improves the body's ability to deal with stress. Add schizandra powder to pancakes, tonics, smoothies, and raw chocolate for an overall beautifying effect.

OTHER HELPFUL FOODS

nettle
Nettle leaves are full of iron and potassium, so a nettle tea or salad is great for treating anemia and is safe even in pregnancy (boil the leaves briefly before eating to take out the sting). Drinking nettle tea and eating the leaves are also said to be helpful in the treatment of asthma and to help regulate blood sugar levels (in conjunction with traditional Western medicine); and a nettle infusion rubbed into the scalp will reduce the oiliness of hair. The root, boiled and drunk, can ease common allergies.

juniper
Juniper is used to treat minor bladder and kidney problems, as well as indigestion, flatulence, and water retention. Usually, the juniper berries are added to a little oil, such as almond or rosehip, and applied to the skin, which also boosts the circulation. The berries taste lovely in vinegar used for pickling vegetables or fish, or to flavor game and stuffing, or even with coleslaw. Don't eat it or use the oil during pregnancy.

camphor
Used as an inhalation, it stimulates the nervous system and circulation (thus used to wake people who have fainted)—and helps relieve menstrual pain. A very diluted camphor compress can also help menstrual pain, and treat chapped lips. A couple of drops of camphor to oil/fat can make a lip balm (see page 109). Do not use the oil undiluted on the skin.

almond
The nut is eaten to ease constipation. Almond milk can be made from ground almonds diluted with water and can be used for babies and adults who are allergic to cow's milk. Almond oil is a great carrier oil for essential oils, particularly for medicinal massages; almond oil alone can help heal rough, chapped, dry, or red skin.

blackberry
Tea made from blackberry root is drunk to treat diarrhea and hemorrhoids, and gargled with to ease sore throats; diluted tea can be used to bathe sore and red eyes. Crushed berries applied to the skin can lessen acne and beautify oily skin, as well as help small open wounds and scratches stop bleeding and close. Young blackberry shoots are eaten as a salad in spring to cure cystitis.

walnut
The outer green skin can be applied directly to the skin to protect wounds, as it contains natural iodine; the skin is also chopped up and eaten to relieve diarrhea and anemia. The nut rubbed on the skin will lessen skin complaints, from eczema and acne to sunburn and chapped lips. To make a natural antiperspirant, boil the leaves of the walnut tree; bathe your feet and hands in the cooled infusion, and dab on the underarm area.

blueberry
Eaten to ward off bladder problems, especially bladder infections, and treat diarrhea. It is said to improve vision when eaten regularly. There is some evidence that it keeps blood pressure and harmful cholesterol low.

hazelnut
This is eaten to strengthen the immune system and get a sluggish digestive system going. Hazelnut also contains lots of B vitamins and potassium.

licorice
Licorice root is chewed to help against a range of lung complaints, from coughs and bronchitis to asthma. It also strengthens the immune system to deal with allergies and after taking strong traditional medicines such as antibiotics and steroids. Licorice is drunk as a strong tea to detoxify. Chewing on licorice can raise your blood pressure briefly, so it should not be taken by those who suffer from high blood pressure.

Due to its strong, sweet flavor, it can be used to mask the bitter taste of other medicinal herbs.

mistletoe

Mistletoe is used with a carrier oil (see page 12) as a rub to treat the symptoms of arthritis. To treat dizziness, it can be drunk as a tea, or added to alcohol (it could be made in advance and carried with you). This plant is somewhat poisonous and should not be ingested unless you are familiar with its properties.

corn

Corn silk (the "hairs" of a sheaf of corn) is boiled and drunk to treat urinary infections and to cure bedwetting in children; it also stimulates the appetite.

celery

A stick of celery can be applied directly to the skin to treat fungal infections. Eaten or drunk as tea, celery will help clear up skin problems and stimulate the circulation and blood flow, such as to bring on menstruation. Celery seeds are sometimes chewed to ease stress and nervousness and may lower blood pressure.

cucumber

Refreshing to the mind and body, cucumber can be applied to sunburnt skin to heal it (see page 36), to bee stings to reduce swelling, and to aching feet to soothe them.

poppy

Boiled in liquid (usually wine), poppy seeds can be drunk to ease stomach upsets. They give great energy and are often eaten by athletes before a long day's training. A syrup or tea can be made from poppy petals to promote sleep.

lemon

A cut lemon rubbed on the skin is used to treat varicose veins and hemorrhoids as well as cellulite. Lemon peel is eaten to ease upset stomachs. Lemon is great for boosting the immune system, especially in winter, due to its high vitamin C content, and lemon diluted in

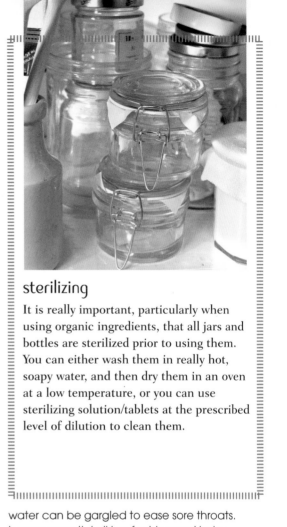

sterilizing

It is really important, particularly when using organic ingredients, that all jars and bottles are sterilized prior to using them. You can either wash them in really hot, soapy water, and then dry them in an oven at a low temperature, or you can use sterilizing solution/tablets at the prescribed level of dilution to clean them.

water can be gargled to ease sore throats. Lemon essential oil is refreshing and helps with concentration—you can use it in an aromatherapy burner.

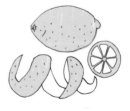

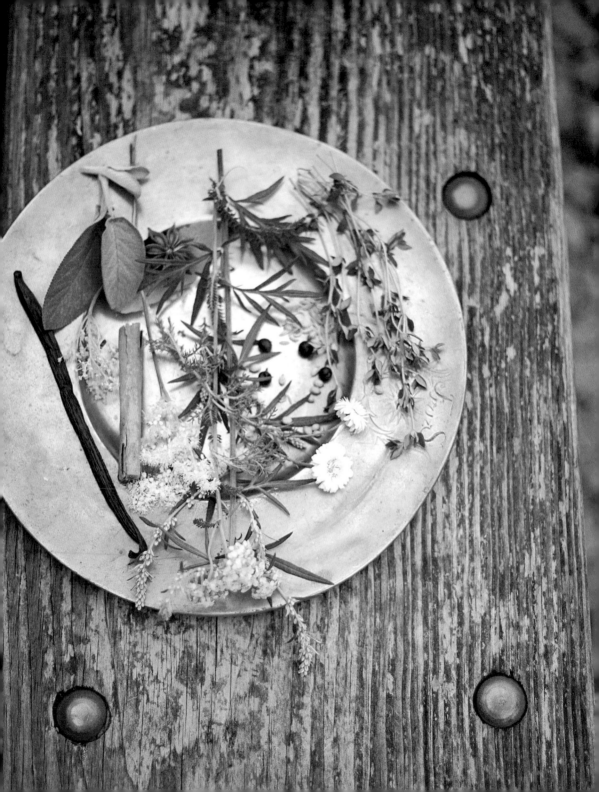

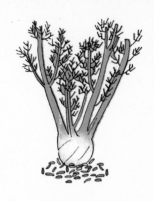

chapter 1

relieving aches, pains, and injuries

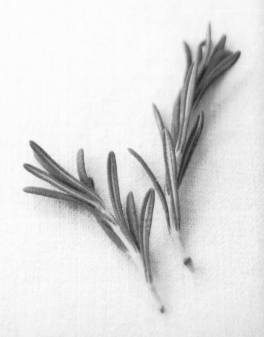

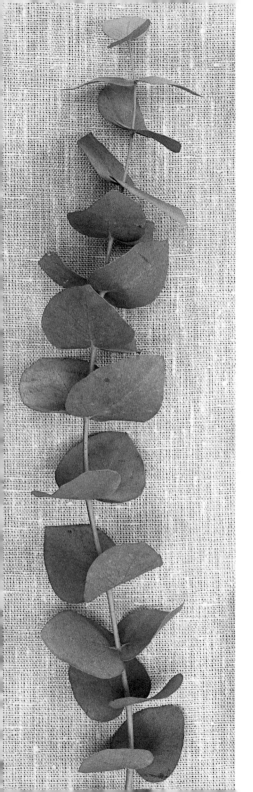

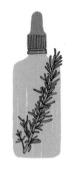

breathe easy salt

Banish colds and coughs or keep them at bay with this sweet-smelling respiratory aid.

10 drops rosemary essential oil
10 drops tea tree essential oil
10 drops eucalyptus essential oil
10 drops lavender essential oil
1 teaspoon sea salt

Shake all the oils and salt together in a small bottle, then hold the open container in both hands under your nose and breathe in deeply three times.

You can also administer this respiratory booster via a vaporizer or bath. Mix the oils only, without the salt, and add four drops to the water of a vaporizer or diffuser or a cotton ball tucked into your pillowcase, or pour six drops into the running water of a hot bath.

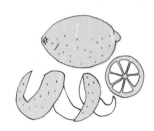

oxymel: an ancient tonic

Oxymel is a very old-fashioned tonic that dates back to ancient times. It remains a favorite of herbal healers and is made of two seemingly opposing ingredients—honey and vinegar. Herbs can be added to great effect and when you see honey-menthol cough drops on the pharmacy shelf, note their 2,000-year-old origins. Oxymels are supremely effective for respiratory issues.

herbs—any from the following: oregano, elder flower, sage, balm,

mint, lemon peel, thyme, lavender, rose petals,

hyssop, or fennel

honey

vinegar

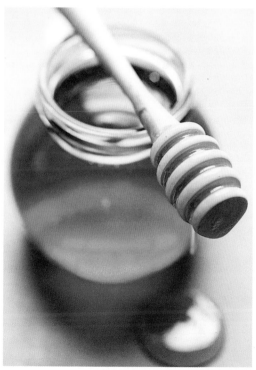

Place your chosen herbs into the canning jar, then pour over equal parts honey and vinegar. Store in a dark cupboard and give the sealed jar a good shake every day. After two weeks, strain out the herbs through cheesecloth and store in the fridge. Drink a tablespoon of tonic for relief from your symptoms. You can also cook with the oxymel or add it to tea.

cough teas

Simple teas can have power healing effects. The two tea recipes below can combat colds and coughs—try both to see which taste you prefer.

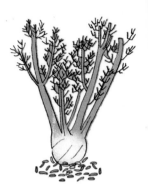

recipe 1

2 oz (50 g) dried sage

2 oz (50 g) dried marjoram

10 star anise

2 oz (50 g) dried coltsfoot

honey or molasses, to taste

recipe 2

2 oz (50 g) dried thyme

2 oz (50 g) dried verbena

2 oz (50 g) dried fennel

2 oz (50 g) dried mullein flowers

honey or molasses, to taste

Mix together all the ingredients. Use three pinches of the mixture for a large cup of tea, add boiling water, and let it steep for five to ten minutes. Strain out the herbs, then sweeten with honey or molasses if desired.

ginger and carrot soup

Ginger is an energetic herb and adds fire and spice to anything it is used for, whether a healing cup of tea, a salad, a savory dish, or this special soup. Ginger root helps to soothe the symptoms of colds, congestion, flu, and fever. Combine it with carrots, which are wonderfully grounding, and you have a simple, comforting soup.

1 lb (450 g) carrots, cleaned and sliced; set aside the carrot greens

4 cups (900 ml) water

1 tablespoon fresh ginger, chopped

1 large garlic clove, peeled and crushed

¼ teaspoon crushed red pepper, plus extra to garnish

½ teaspoon salt

1 lemon

Serves 6

Put the carrots in a big pot and add the water. Bring to a boil, then simmer on a medium heat for 20–25 minutes, adding the ginger, garlic, red pepper, and salt after 5 minutes.

When the carrots are tender, transfer them with their water to a blender and blend until smooth. Stir in several squeezes of lemon juice and pour into bowls or mugs. Garnish with a few chopped carrot greens and a sprinkling of crushed red pepper.

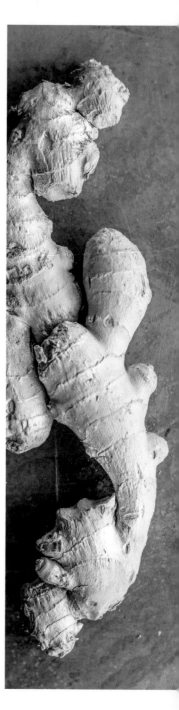

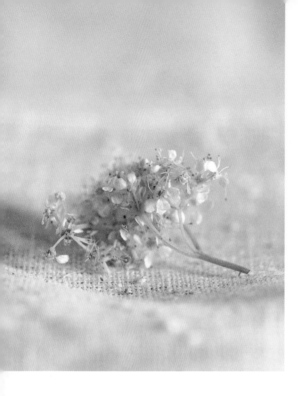

fever tea

This tea helps break a fever, ease rheumatism, and strengthen the constitution after an illness.

¾ oz (20 g) dried thyme flowers
¾ oz (20 g) dried holly leaves
¾ oz (20 g) dried elder flowers
¾ oz (20 g) dried lime flowers
¾ oz (20 g) dried meadowsweet
honey or molasses, to taste

Mix together all the ingredients. Use about three pinches to make a large cup of tea. Infuse in boiling water and strain off the herbs. Sweeten with honey or molasses if desired.

soothing stomach tea

This is the perfect tea to settle a bloated, painful stomach.

2 oz (50 g) dried peppermint
2 oz (50 g) dried chamomile
¾ oz (20 g) dried wormwood
pinch caraway seeds

Mix all the ingredients together. Use about three pinches to make a large cup of tea; infuse in boiling water and strain off the herbs. It is best not to use sweetener to ensure this tea can work its best.

blackberry tonic for tummy aches and cramps

Blackberries are one of life's sweetest gifts, growing abundantly in the bramble along rambling paths. This tonic is so powerful that you can add a teaspoon into a cup of water and cure tummy aches, cramps, fevers, coughs, and colds.

4 cups (520 g) blackberries
1 quart (1 liter) malt vinegar
about 4½ cups sugar (see recipe)

Soaking the berries in the vinegar for three days. Drain and strain the liquid into a pan. Simmer and stir in the sugar, 2¼ cups (450 g) to every 2 cups (475 ml) of tonic. Boil gently for 5 minutes and skim off any foam. Cool and pour into a sealable jar.

it's delicious, too!

As well as being a medicine, blackberry vinegar is a highly prized culinary flavoring for sauces and salads. Pour some over your apple pie and cream and you will soon scurry off to pick blackberries all summer.

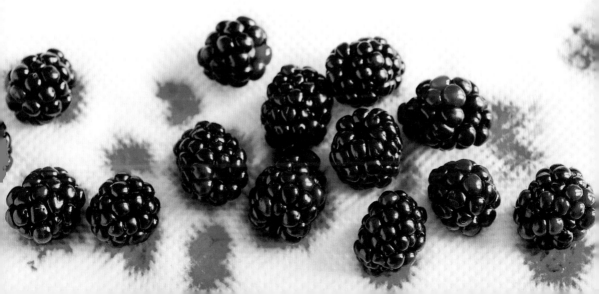

ways to relieve digestive discomfort

If your stomach is feeling a little off, whether from overindulging or having eaten something that disagreed with you, there are a number of natural ways to settle it and restore a feeling of balance.

walking

Take a gentle walk after eating a meal. A short walk around the block will rev your metabolism, add an element of mobility, and break up heaviness from overeating. Don't go for a run—the aim is to get things moving in a downward flow, not to sweat out any toxins you've just eaten. You can save your sweat for a day later.

herbal formula

Triphala is an herbal formula that is a natural, rejuvenating detoxifier and purifier that is good to take nightly and it can also be handy to take when you have overindulged. Triphala is made of three herbs: amalaka, bibhitaki, and haritaki. It promotes healthy weight loss and it also tones, nourishes, and strengthens the entire body. If taken after a meal, triphala will give your body a gentle cleanse, help remove any lingering toxicity formed by the food, and reset your digestion so you feel ready to go the next day.

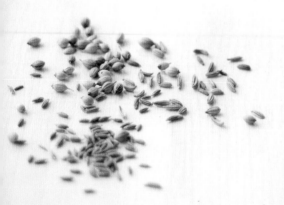

the fennel trick

At one time or another, most of us have eaten too much in one meal and instantly felt bloated. Luckily, there is an easy fix for a stuffed and bloated tummy: fennel. One of the simplest ways to incorporate it into your diet is to chew about twenty fennel seeds after a meal. Fennel helps to digest heavy sauces and carb-centric dishes, which is why you often see a bowl of fennel seeds at the exit of Indian restaurants. Drinking warm water will also help lessen the bloat.

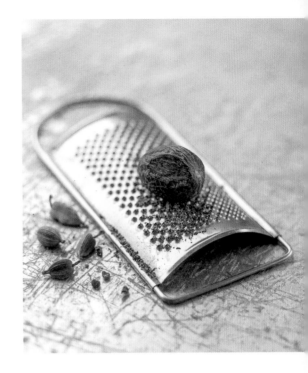

nutmeg milk

Grated nutmeg soothes heartburn, nausea, and upset tummies. Use a grater to grate a small amount (about ⅛ teaspoon) to 1 mug of warmed milk (cow, soy, rice, or oat milk). It is comforting and curing.

catnip tea

This herb is not just for kitties! We humans can also benefit from it as a remedy for upset tummies as well as a way to diminish worry, anxiety, and nervous tension. Take a palmful of dried catnip leaves and steep in a cup (240 ml) of boiling water for 5 minutes. Strain as you would any loose tea. Honey helps even more and a cup or two of catnip tea per day will have you in fine fettle, relaxed and ready.

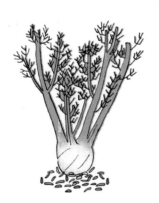

gripe water

This is great for relieving trapped wind. Boil 18 fl oz (500 ml) water and pour over 1 teaspoon each of dill and crushed fennel seeds. Let this infuse for 20 minutes. Strain out the seeds. Add just under 1 oz (20 g) brown sugar if desired, and make sure it dissolves completely. The mixture can be stored in the fridge for a couple of days and should be drunk at room temperature.

red clover lemonade

The beautiful flowers of red clover are slightly sweet, and many of us will have enjoyed them in clover honey. They are also packed with nutrients, calcium, magnesium, potassium, and vitamin C. Red clover has been used in tea form for many years to alleviate the symptoms of gout. This lemonade is a quick and easy recipe that leaves you with a very pretty, delicately flavored sweet drink—think sweet hay.

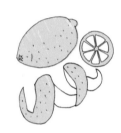

3 cups (750 ml) water

Approximately 40 red clover blossoms

1 cup (250 ml) freshly squeezed lemon juice

3 tablespoons (50 ml) honey, preferably raw, set or runny

Soda water

Serves 6 (approximately 1 quart/1 liter)

Bring the water to a slow boil in a small, nonreactive pan, add the clover blossoms, and gently simmer for 5 minutes. Strain the liquid into a wide-mouthed pitcher, removing the blossoms, and return to the cleaned pan over a low heat. Add the lemon juice and honey, and stir to dissolve the honey. Do not let it boil. Remove from the heat and pour the lemonade into the cleaned pitcher. Chill for a couple of hours in the refrigerator. To serve, fill the 6 glasses with ice. Pour the lemonade three-quarters of the way up each one. Garnish with fresh red clover blossoms. Top with soda water and serve immediately.

properties of red clover

Coumarin, the phytochemical present in red clover, has antifungal and antitumor properties, but it also thins the blood. While that may be great for some, people taking anticoagulants should not consume red clover in large quantities.

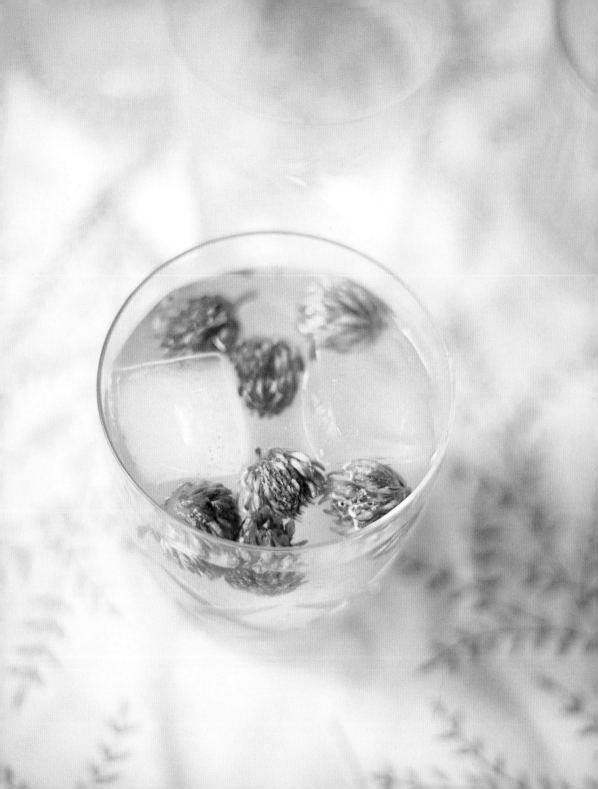

gardener's tea for aching joints

Harvesting herbs and veggies and weeding is a huge amount of work. It is one of life's greatest joys, without doubt, but nevertheless, many a sore back and aching knees have come as result of a thriving garden. This tea revives, refreshes, and offers relief to aching joints.

2 parts dried echinacea
2 parts dried chamomile
1 part dried mint
1 part anise seed
1 part dried thyme

Gather the ingredients from your store of dried herbs and add boiling water. Allow to steep, then strain into a cup. A nice hot cup of this remedy will have you jumping back into the garden to plant more of all the herbs that comprise this delightful tea.

thyme tincture for sore muscles

Wherever thyme goes, it fills the air with its magnificent scent and elegant beauty. If possible, keep a plenitude growing and several bunches drying in a dark corner of your pantry at all times as this plant makes a mighty fine tincture with many medicinal uses.

1¼ cups (65 g) dried thyme leaves
2 cups (480 ml) apple cider vinegar

Put the dried thyme inside a 17-fl oz (500-ml) jar and carefully pour the vinegar inside. Stir well and seal. Place on a dark shelf and shake it every day. At the end of the one month, strain through muslin, and store the remaining tincture in another jar. (The thyme residue can be composted in your garden.)

Simply rub a little of the tincture wherever you have aches and pains for instant relief.

To enjoy a cup of thyme tea, add one teaspoon of the tincture into a cup of hot water, add a teaspoon of honey and stir.

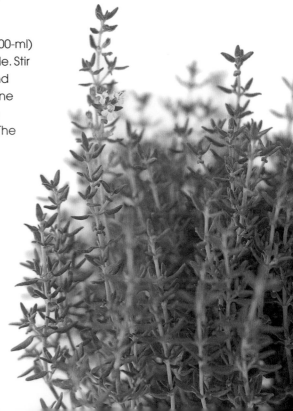

peppermint oil for muscular pain

To relieve sore muscles, massage the affected area with peppermint oil. If you use a commercial oil, check that it is suitable for external use.

oregano and allspice healing bath

Relieve aches and pains with this delightful bath infusion.

oregano

allspice

cheesecloth

Place the oregano and allspice in the middle of the cheesecloth. Tie the four corners of the cloth to make a pouch. Run a warm bath and place the pouch into the bath water. As you get into the bath, imagine yourself encased in a bubble of healing. When you are ready to get out of the bath, open the spice pouch, then take the plug out of the bath. Watch the water and spices drain down the plughole and as you do so, imagine all the sickness, pain, and discomfort leaving your body.

lavender to help headaches

Lavender is hard not to grow, and once your seedlings and young plants have been established, they will bush out and produce loads of scented stalks, flowers, and seeds. This bounty will become your source for teas, tinctures, bath salts, and infusions.

lavender tea

For tea, the rule of thumb is 1 teaspoon dried lavender flowers to 1 cup (240 ml) boiling water to aid headaches and calm the mind, as well as to help with tummy trouble, aches, and insomnia. You can easily amp up the therapeutic power of your brew, by adding dried yarrow, St. John's wort, or chamomile.

lavender infusion

This is a simple and streamlined way to infuse lavender. Pour a heaping tablespoon of lavender into a bowl of hot water and then drape a towel over your head and breathe in the aromatic fumes to deal with headaches and nervous tension. It can also ease respiratory issues, coughs, colds, and stuffy sinuses. You will come away feeling renewed and your kitchen will smell like the heavens above. You can use the water in your morning bath or add to your sink garbage disposal—grinding up the flowers refreshes that hard-duty kitchen appliance.

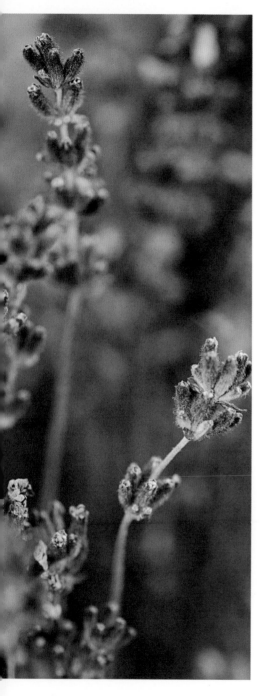

lavender tincture

This cure-all can be kept on hand at all times for soothing the skin, the stomach, and anything in need of comfort. I have even seen it used to staunch bleeding in small cuts.

dried lavender

1 cup (240 ml) clear alcohol, such as vodka

2 cups (480 ml) distilled water

Fill a clear quart jar to the halfway point with the dried lavender. Pour in the alcohol also to the halfway point. Add in the water, seal securely with a lid, and shake for a few minutes until it seems well mixed. Store in a dark cupboard for one month, shaking once a day. After 30 days, strain through a cheesecloth into a dark glass storage jar and screw the lid on tightly. The liquid tincture will soon prove itself indispensable in your household, and the strained out lavender will make lovely compost.

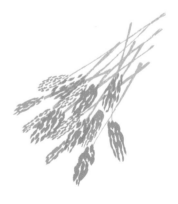

comfrey and lavender cure-all salve

Comfrey is one of the best-known healing herbs of all times. Well known and widely used by early Greeks and Romans, its botanical name, symphytum, from the Greek "symphyo," means to "make grow together," referring to its traditional use of healing fractures. Comfrey relieves pain and inflammation, so comfrey salve will be a mainstay of your home first-aid kit. Use it on cuts, scrapes, rashes, sunburn, and almost any skin irritation. It can also bring comfort to aching arthritic joints and sore muscles.

¾ cup (180 ml) comfrey-infused oil

¼ cup (60 ml) coconut oil

4 tablespoons beeswax

10 drops lavender essential oil

Combine the comfrey and coconut oils. Heat the oil and wax together until the wax melts completely. Pour into a clean, dry jar. When the mixture has cooled a little, but not yet set, add 10 drops of lavender essential oil, which is also an antiseptic. Stir it through.

Seal the jar and store in a cabinet to use anytime you scratch yourself working in the garden or want to renew and soften your hands and feet after a lot of house and yard work.

Please note: use the salve only on the outside of your skin—if a cut is deep, don't let it get inside the wound.

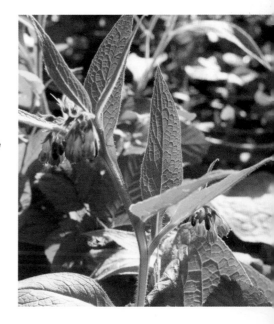

cucumber lotion

Homegrown, organic cucumber makes a deliciously cool lotion, especially for the face—marvelous for hot summer days. It's also very soothing when applied to sunburned skin. Keep a bottle of the lotion in the fridge and use within two weeks.

> fresh cucumber
>
> eau de cologne, optional

Coarsely grate the cucumber and place in a sieve lined with fine cheesecloth. Place the sieve over a bowl and push the cucumber through the cheesecloth to release the juice. Pour the resulting liquid into a clean glass jar or spray bottle. Add a few drops of eau de cologne for a scented lotion, and apply as required.

other skin solutions

Try these other natural cures for burned or irritated skin.

SAGE: To make a lotion for sunburned skin, tear a handful of fresh sage leaves into a bowl, cover with boiling water and infuse for 20 minutes. Strain into a bottle, refrigerate, and apply when needed.

SAINT-JOHN'S-WORT: The mashed yellow flowers of Saint-John's-Wort mixed with olive oil make a soothing lotion for sunburn or varicose veins.

ALOE VERA: As a topical application, aloe-vera gel is great for all kinds of burns, and it has been shown to have therapeutic value in the healing of skin lesions caused by psoriasis. To use for a burn, bug bite, rash, scratch, itch, or sunburn, simply grab a stem and apply the juice liberally to the affected area. You can also make batches of aloe gel. All you do is gather and wash the leaves, peel the skin, and harvest the gel inside. You can store it in the refrigerator for ten days.

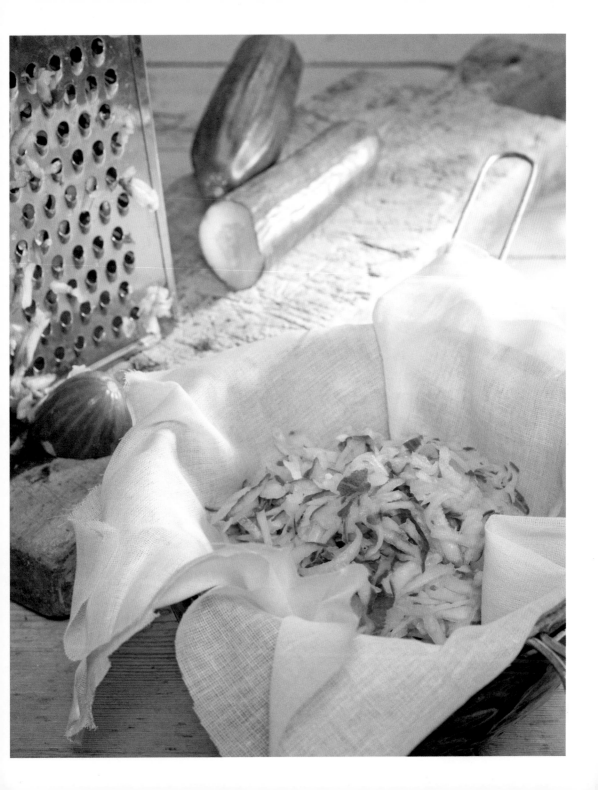

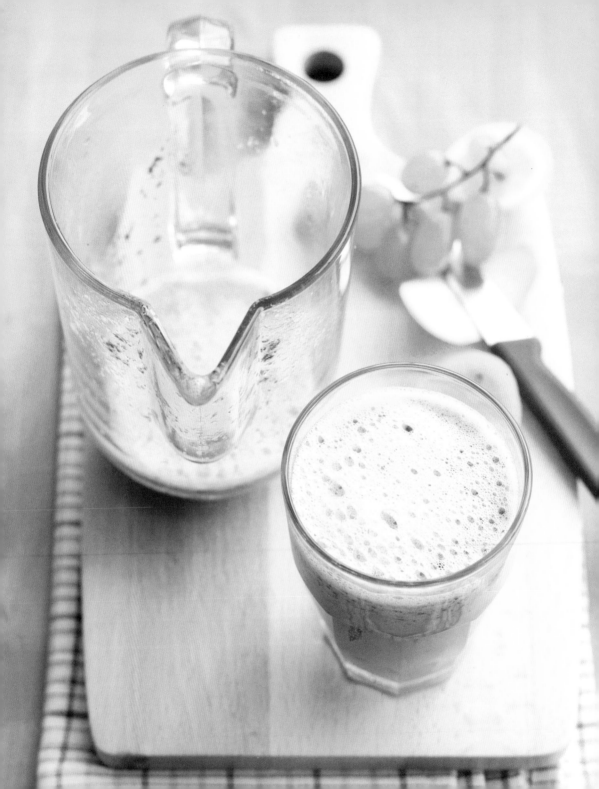

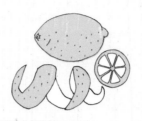

chapter 2

maintaining good health

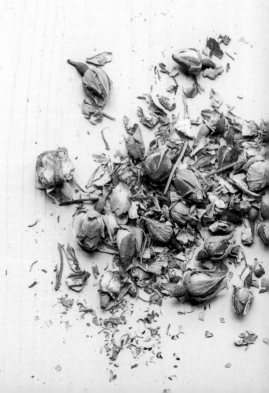

vitamin C tea

This tonic provides bioflavonoids and vitamin C in an organic, natural way so all the nutrients are easily available for absorption. The amounts of ingredients are given in parts, so you can make a big batch of tea for the whole family.

2 parts lemongrass
3 parts hibiscus
4 parts rose hips
1 part chopped cinnamon sticks
4 cups (960 ml) hot water
honey

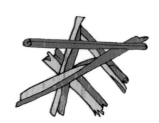

Blend the herbs using a mortar and pestle. Place in a teapot with the hot water. Steep for 5 minutes in your teapot, then strain and serve sweetened with honey to taste. If you make ahead, you should keep the mixed herbs in an airtight container. Serve regularly as a preventative during cold and flu season.

rose hip tea

Ground rose hips contain 50 percent more immune-boosting Vitamin C than oranges. One tablespoon provides more than the recommended daily adult allowance of 90 mg for men and 75 mg for women.

1 oz (28 g) dried rosehips
1 oz (28 g) dried hibiscus
2 oz (56 g) dried mint
1 tablespoon dried ginger root

Place all the ingredients together in a teapot and stir to mix. Pour hot water over the herbs, two teaspoons per cup, and let steep for 5 minutes.

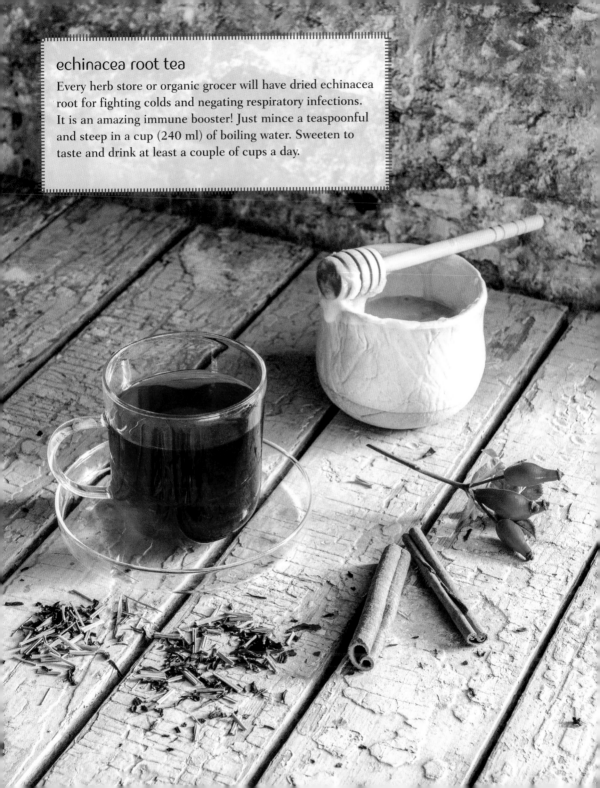

echinacea root tea

Every herb store or organic grocer will have dried echinacea root for fighting colds and negating respiratory infections. It is an amazing immune booster! Just mince a teaspoonful and steep in a cup (240 ml) of boiling water. Sweeten to taste and drink at least a couple of cups a day.

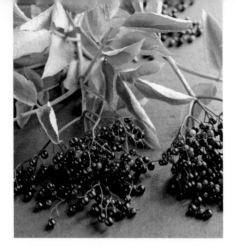

elderberry flu buster

Elderberries are said to boost the immune system, have antioxidant properties, improve heart health, and tackle viral infections, because bioflavonoids and other proteins in the juice destroy the ability of cold and flu viruses to infect a cell. They are high in vitamin C, potassium, beta carotene, calcium, and phosphorus. Cloves make an ideal pairing, reducing inflammation and aiding digestion. You could serve this hot with slices of fresh ginger to open up the sinuses.

2 oz (60 ml) Elderberry and Clove Syrup (see opposite)

1 oz (30 ml) Ginger Syrup (see opposite)

1 teaspoon (10 ml) raw, set honey

6 oz (180 ml) boiling water

spear of freshly peeled ginger

Serves 1

Measure the syrups and honey into a mug or a heatproof glass. Pour boiling water almost to the top and stir hard until all the ingredients are combined. Garnish with a spear of fresh ginger.

elderberry and clove syrup

25 heads of elderberries

at least 4 cups (1 liter) water

3¼ cups (750 g) superfine (caster) sugar

12 cloves

Makes approximately 1 quart (1 liter)

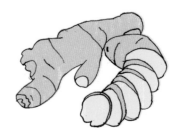

Strip the berries from the stems using your fingers or a fork. (Elderberry stems and stalks are poisonous, and even the berries are slightly toxic if eaten raw in quantity, so make sure you strip the berries from the stalks and don't be tempted to munch on them.) Rinse the berries, then add to a nonreactive pan. Pour in enough water to cover them (at least 1 quart/1 liter). Bring to a boil and let simmer on a low heat until the berries are softened (about 20 minutes).

Mash the berries gently to ensure all the juice has been released. Remove from the heat and strain the berries into a wide-mouthed measuring cup. You should have just over 1 quart (1 liter) of juice. Add the sugar and cloves. Return the liquid, sugar, and cloves to the cleaned pan and bring to a boil. Let simmer for a further 10 minutes. Remove from the heat and funnel into a sterilized presentation bottle (see page 17). Divide the cloves up equally between the bottles and seal.

Store in a cool, dark place, where the syrup will last for up to a year. Once opened, keep in the refrigerator for up to 2 months. You may wish to remove the cloves after a time if their flavor becomes too strong.

ginger syrup

2 cups (400 g) superfine (caster) sugar

2 cups (500 ml) water

2½ oz (75 g) fresh ginger, fairly thickly sliced

1 tablespoon lemon juice (optional)

Makes approximately 1 pint (500 ml)

Place the sugar and water in a nonreactive pan and slowly bring to a boil. Add the ginger and let simmer for 5 minutes. Remove from the heat and let the ginger steep for another 10 minutes.

Strain the syrup into a wide-mouthed pitcher and then funnel into a sterilized presentation bottle (see page 17) and seal. Store in the refrigerator and consume within 2 weeks. A tablespoon of lemon juice added just after removing the pan from the heat will increase the shelf life of the syrup for up to a month.

lavender and honey mocktail

It is claimed that local raw honey can help hay fever sufferers develop an immunity to the local pollen. Raw honey is also rich in cancer-fighting phytonutrients and powerful antioxidants which are found in the propolis that the bees use to sterilize the beehive. The acacia blossoms provide extra floral notes but aren't strictly necessary. As well as being good for you, this summer mocktail punch tastes delicious. You can make it in quantity in advance and then top up everyone's glass with soda water on the day.

2 cups (640 g) raw, runny honey

2 cups (500 ml) warm water

2 heaped tablespoons fresh edible-grade lavender buds
or 4 teaspoons dried lavender blossoms (see box)

2 heads of acacia blossom (optional, if in season)

1 cup (250 ml) freshly squeezed lemon juice

2 lemons, sliced into thin wheels

1 cup (20 g) lemon balm (Melissa officinalis) or mint (Mentha) leaves

splash of soda water

lavender sprigs

lemon balm sprigs

Serves 6 (makes approximately 1½ pints (750ml)

Combine the honey and water in a large nonreactive pan and stir over a low heat until the honey liquefies and dissolves. Just before the liquid boils, add the lavender buds and acacia blossom heads (if you have them), remove the pan from the heat, and let steep for 20 minutes.

Strain the mixture using a fine-strainer or cheesecloth into a large pitcher to remove the lavender buds (and blossoms). Return the liquid to the cleaned pan, then add the lemon juice and the lemon wheels. Smack the lemon balm or mint leaves between your palms to release the essential oils. Add to the pan. Let stand for an hour.

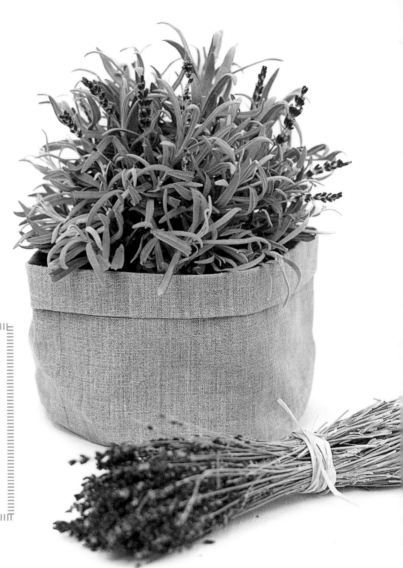

If you wish, strain the mocktail punch again. Alternatively, remove the lemon balm or mint leaves and serve using a ladle. Fill 6 glasses with ice. Pour the punch two-thirds of the way up each glass. Top with a splash of soda water. Garnish with the sprig of lavender and fresh sprigs of mint or lemon balm.

sleep tea

This tea will help you go to sleep after a stressful day or when suffering from insomnia.

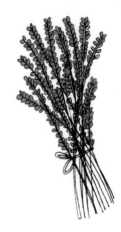

 2 oz (50 g) dried elder flowers
 2 oz (50 g) dried lavender
 2 oz (50 g) dried hawthorn flowers
 2 oz (50 g) dried hops flowers
 2 oz (50 g) dried valerian leaves
 2 oz (50 g) dried basil leaves

Mix everything together. Use about three pinches to make a large cup of tea; infuse in boiling water and strain off the herbs. Drink about 45 minutes prior to bedtime.

sleep milk

Pair this tonic with a warm bath or sleep ritual to enhance the dreamy vibes. The ghee is grounding and nourishing, which is perfect right before sleep.

 1 teaspoon ghee
 ½ tablespoon ashwagandha powder
 ½ tablespoon mucuna pruriens powder
 ½ teaspoon astragalus powder
 1½ cups (350 ml) warm almond milk (or other nut milk)
 1 teaspoon raw honey

Serves 1

Heat the ghee in a saucepan over a low heat for 1 minute, then add the herbs and simmer for 30 seconds. Add the milk and stir. (If you have a hand-held milk frother or whisk, you may use it to froth the milk.) Remove from the heat. Once the liquid has cooled to a warm temperature, add the honey.

herbal helpers

Try these other simple sleep solutions for a good night's rest.

hops

As we all know, hops are used for beer-making but did you know that, in the form of a tincture, they excel as a sleeping aid and stress-reliever? Women healers claim that hops are very useful to calm hot flashes in menopause. The ideal dosage of 2–4 ml before sleep is said to help anxiety.

valerian root

Valerian, native to Europe and North America, has long been used to treat anxiety, stress, muscle tension, and insomnia. It contains valerenic acid and valeranon, which help the body relax into a calm state so that sleep can come naturally. You can either chop fresh valerian root with your bolline or use the dried version, which is easily obtained in herb stores. Use the same recipe as for skullcap tincture (see page 83), replacing the skullcap with valerian root, for a dreamy sleep potion that will relax you, body and soul.

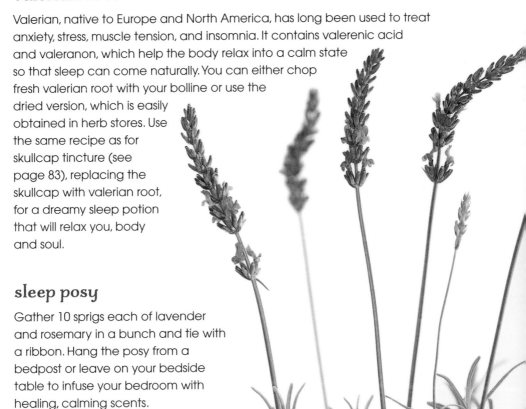

sleep posy

Gather 10 sprigs each of lavender and rosemary in a bunch and tie with a ribbon. Hang the posy from a bedpost or leave on your bedside table to infuse your bedroom with healing, calming scents.

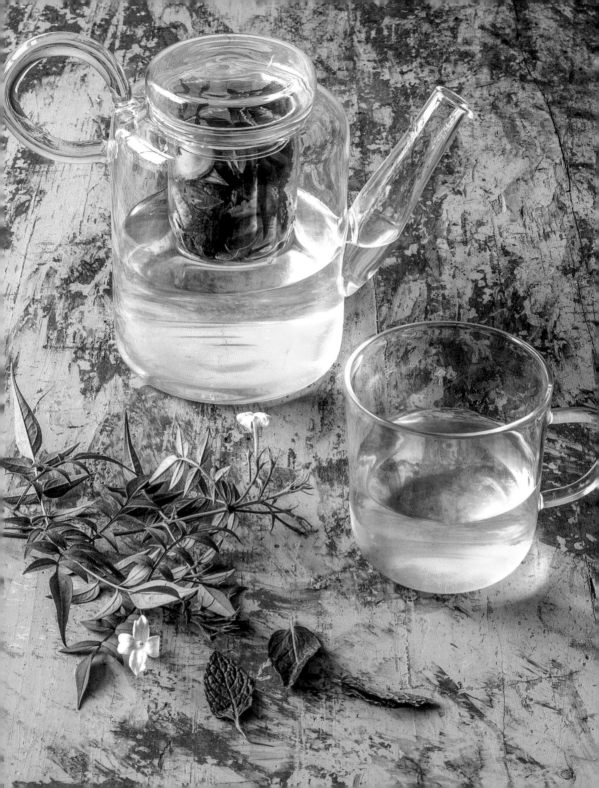

restorative infusion for energy

Try this restorative elixir anytime your energy level is low to bolster mind, body, and spirit.

- 1 teaspoon sliced fresh ginger root
- 1 teaspoon jasmine tea leaves
- 1 teaspoon peppermint tea leaves
- 2 cups (480 ml) hot water

Place the ginger, jasmine, and peppermint in a pan and add the hot water. Let brew for 5 minutes, then strain and pour into a mug.

apple cider vinegar

Apple cider vinegar lowers cholesterol and blood pressure and helps strengthen bones. Here's how to make your own.

- 8 organic apple cores and peels
- 1 quart (1 liter) water
- 2 tablespoons honey

Cut up the apple cores and peels into smaller pieces and spoon into a wide-mouthed canning jar. Pour in the water to cover the fruit, spoon in the honey, and stir well. Cover the mixture with a clean paper towel or waxed paper and place a rubber band tightly around the neck of the jar. Place on a dark shelf in your cupboard or work area and leave for two weeks.

Strain the liquid and remove the compostable solids that remain, return the liquid to the jar and secure the paper and band again. Put it back on the shelf and make sure to stir daily. After one month, take a spoonful and if the acidity and flavor is to your taste, transfer to a dark bottle with sealable top. If not, wait another week and then taste it again. Vinegar will corrode metal lids so a bottle with a cork is the best option.

Drink one or two teaspoons of apple cider vingear a day, or make use of it in salad dressings and other recipes to gain its health benefits.

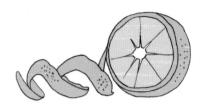

vitali-tea

This is a great tea to enjoy when you need to detox. The liver and kidneys play an important role in keeping our bodies clean. When we support these two organs, we are aiding the body in the process of detoxification. Dandelion root is one of the best remedies for supporting the liver. It is also revered as a diuretic and can help reduce water retention. Licorice root supports the digestive system and helps push extra toxins out of our organs. Cinnamon and cardamom are warming, and orange peel is slightly heating and super rich in vitamin C.

1 tablespoon licorice root

1 tablespoon dandelion root

½ tablespoon dried orange peel

½ teaspoon cardamom seeds

¼ teaspoon cinnamon chips

2 cups (475 ml) boiled water

raw honey, to taste

Serves 2

Put the herbs and boiled water in a bowl and let the mixture steep for 20 minutes. (Since we are working with roots, its best to let the tea steep for longer than we do when making teas with leaves or flowers.) Using a strainer or cheesecloth (muslin), strain the tea and pour into a thermos. Once the tea has cooled to a warm temperature, add the raw honey and enjoy!

dandelion, sassafras and ginger detox

Sassafras was highly prized by Native Americans who used it for medicine and were extremely knowledgeable about combining herbs to amplify their power. This morning tonic is inspired by a shamanic native-healing recipe. It is pleasantly surprising how good the detox tastes and even more how the herbs combine to eliminate toxins from the body, chiefly the kidney and liver. After over-indulging, this purifying herbal blend will cleanse the organs that cleanse your body, thus aiding wellness. This detox should be used seasonally and is not intended for daily use, due to its great power.

½ cup sassafras roots
½ cup dandelion greens
½ cup wild ginger, sliced
honey, to taste

To make this wonderfully medicinal decoction, combine the ingredients and boil them in spring water. After steeping for 12 minutes, strain, stir in honey as desired, and enjoy.

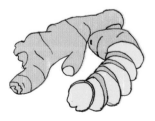

birch, ginger, and wisteria detoxer

This mocktail is a great detoxer. Sap from the white birch (Betula alba) or silver birch (Betula pendula) is one of the healthiest juices you can drink. Unless you know how to harvest it yourself, online is your best place to source it. Unusually, it tackles the body's two cleansing and purification systems—the liver and kidneys—at the same time, and helps flush out harmful toxins, uric acid, and excess water from the body. Its partner here is flavorsome ginger, which fires up the digestive juices and, according to Ayurvedic texts, the libido! Meanwhile, the wisteria flower garnish has a role here primarily for its looks—it's really pretty and the perfect blowzy opposite to the restrained, cloudy-looking tonic. It's also edible.

3 oz (90 ml) birch sap

1 oz (30 ml) Ginger Syrup (see page 43)

¾ oz (22 ml) freshly squeezed lemon juice

splash of soda water

wisteria blossom

Serves 1

Chill a glass thoroughly in the freezer or refrigerator for 2 or 4 hours respectively. Alternatively, fill the glass with ice. Pour all the ingredients into a cocktail shaker and fill it two-thirds of the way up with ice. Cover and shake hard for 20 seconds. If you used ice to chill your glass, empty it out. Strain the cocktail into the glass. Garnish with the wisteria blossom and top with a splash of soda water.

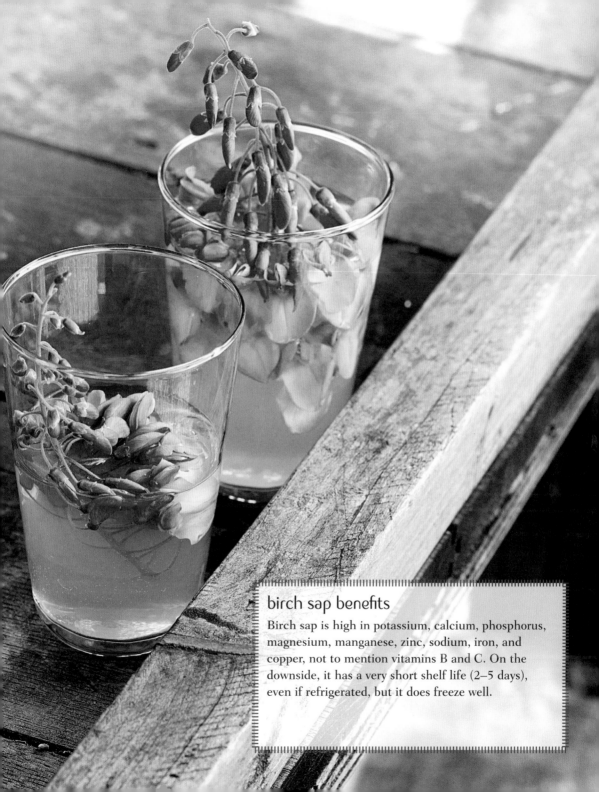

birch sap benefits

Birch sap is high in potassium, calcium, phosphorus, magnesium, manganese, zinc, sodium, iron, and copper, not to mention vitamins B and C. On the downside, it has a very short shelf life (2–5 days), even if refrigerated, but it does freeze well.

fennel, ginger, and lemon thyme reviver

Fennel can help improve the function of a poor, overworked, toxin-laden liver. It's also been called the pearl of aphrodisiacs, so it might really perk you up! Ginger should help wake up your senses and overcome nausea. Thyme helps soothe muscles and stomach at the same time.

1 teaspoon fennel seeds

1 thumbnail-sized piece of ginger, thinly sliced or grated

3 x 3-in (8-cm) long lemon thyme sprigs

boiling water

1 tsp honey, preferably raw, set or runny

thyme sprig

spear of freshly peeled ginger

fennel floret

Serves 1

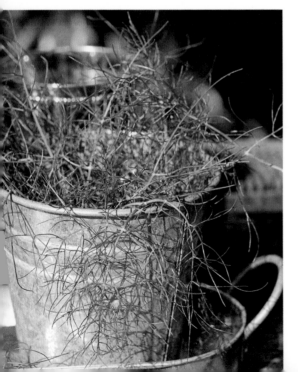

Place the fennel seeds, ginger, and sprigs of lemon thyme in the cup or heatproof glass. Pour over boiling water, almost to the top. Add the honey and stir. Garnish with a thyme sprig, ginger spear, and fennel floret.

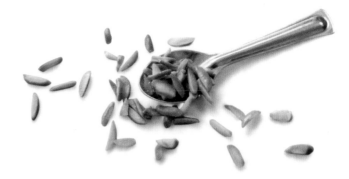

gentle detox tea

This age-old Ayurvedic recipe works wonders if you have been indulging a little too much while on vacation or are battling a post-pizza party belly. The fennel reduces bloating, the cumin helps to balance blood sugar, the coriander acts as a calming agent, and the manjistha is anti-inflammatory and clears the lymphatic system. Drink this tea daily if you're struggling regularly with constant gas, bloating, indigestion, acid reflux, or sluggish digestion. Daily use of this tea will not only promote a gentle full body detox but also facilitate fat burning and aid in the digestion of proteins.

4–5 cups (950 ml–1.2 liters) water

½ teaspoon cumin seeds

½ teaspoon coriander seeds

½ teaspoon fennel seeds

½ teaspoon manjistha powder

Serves 4

Put the water in a saucepan and bring to the boil. Add the remaining ingredients, cover, and let boil for 5 minutes. Using a strainer or cheesecloth (muslin), strain the tea and pour into a thermos. Take small sips of the tea throughout the day or drink 1 cup (250 ml) of the tea before or after meals.

celery juice elixir

Drinking celery juice on an empty stomach helps to produce the stomach acid HCL, which breaks down proteins in the gut, restores electrolyte balance, detoxes the liver and kidneys, hydrates the skin, and lowers blood pressure. Celery is also an excellent source of natural sodium, which can help beat salty cravings when consumed daily.

1 bunch of celery, chopped

1 lemon, halved and peeled

Serves 1

Juice the celery and lemon. Alternatively, if you don't have a juicer, put the celery and lemon in a food processor or blender and blend on a high speed until well blended, then use a nut bag or cheesecloth (muslin) to strain the juice. Drink on an empty stomach for most benefit. The elixir will keep for up to 2 days in an airtight container or jar in the refrigerator.

water and lemon digestion aid

This should be drunk first thing in the morning to cleanse your bowels, promote digestion, and remove toxins.

1 lemon

1½–3¾ cups (350–900 ml) water

½-inch (1-cm) piece of fresh ginger, grated (optional)

1 teaspoon raw honey (optional)

Serves 1

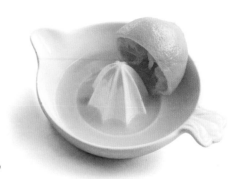

Wash the lemon and then either juice half of it or cut the lemon in half and squeeze some juice into a large mug. Add the rest of the lemon to the mug. Put the water in a small saucepan with the ginger, if using. Heat the water until you see little bubbles forming at the bottom of the pan—do not let the water boil. Pour the warm water into the mug with the lemon juice. Alternatively, if you don't have access to a stovetop, feel free to use a microwave. Heat the water in a microwave-safe cup (ceramic is preferred) in 30-second increments. Heating the water in a microwave for 40–50 seconds will usually warm the water to an enjoyable temperature. If desired, add the raw honey to the finished drink when it has cooled to a warm temperature.

digestive rose tea

The cardamom in this recipe enhances digestion while also calming indigestion and heartburn. The fennel is a potent digestive aid and works wonders in combination with fresh ginger, which is an all-round healer. When ginger is taken before meals it aids in the absorption of nutrients. The rose is cooling and calming in nature, which makes it the perfect partner to balance out these other heating herbs. Rose is rich in vitamin C and revered as a beauty herb.

4–5 cups (950 ml–1.2 liters) water

½ teaspoon cardamom pods

½ teaspoon fennel seeds

¼-inch (5-mm) piece of fresh ginger, peeled and chopped

½ teaspoon dried rose buds

Serves 4

Put the water in a saucepan and bring to the boil. Add all the remaining ingredients, cover, and let boil for 5 minutes. Using a strainer or cheesecloth (muslin), strain the tea and pour into a thermos. Enjoy the tea with snacks or drink it throughout the day for a calming digestive tonic.

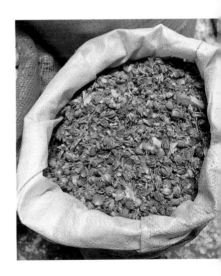

modern kitchari reset

Sometimes we can overload our system and no remedy seems to help. Kitchari can help give your digestive system a break and reset your body back to balance. It is an easy-to-digest complete food and can be eaten every day if you enjoy it. If liked, you can serve this dish topped with your favorite steamed veggies.

2 tablespoons coconut oil

1½ teaspoons cumin seeds

1½ teaspoons fennel seeds

½ teaspoon fenugreek seeds

¼ teaspoon black mustard seeds

1½ teaspoons ground coriander

1 tablespoon minced fresh ginger

½ teaspoon turmeric powder

pinch of asafetida (hing)

4 cups (950 ml) vegetable stock or water

½ cup (100 g) split yellow mung beans, soaked overnight in a bowl of purified water and then drained and rinsed

½ cup (85 g) sprouted quinoa, rinsed

1-inch (2.5-cm) strip of kombu

sea salt

½ cup (25 g) chopped cilantro (fresh coriander)

1 lime, cut into wedges

Serves 4

Heat the coconut oil in a heavy-bottomed saucepan over a medium heat, then add the cumin, fennel, fenugreek, and mustard seeds and cook for a few minutes to release the aromatics, until the mustard seeds start to pop. Add the remaining spices and stir to combine. Add 1 cup (250 ml) of the vegetable stock or water, followed by the mung beans, quinoa, and kombu, then add the remainder of the stock or water. Cover and bring to a boil, then reduce the heat to a simmer and cook for 40 minutes or until the beans and quinoa are tender and the mixture has thickened to a porridge consistency, checking from time to time to make sure the quinoa does not stick to the bottom of the pan. Season with salt. (If you prefer a soupier consistency, add some extra water and simmer for longer to get a thicker stew.) Divide the kitchari between bowls and garnish with cilantro (fresh coriander) and lime wedges to squeeze over. The kitchari will keep for up to 4 days in an airtight container in the refrigerator.

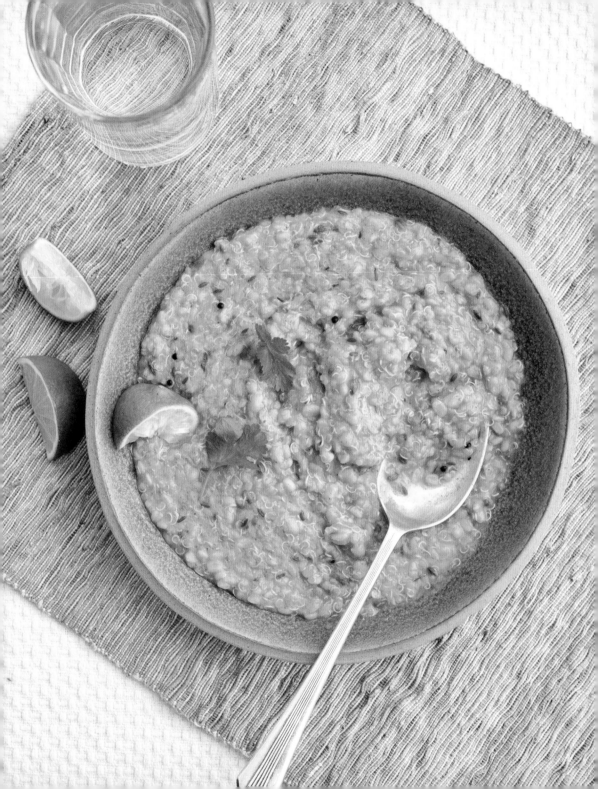

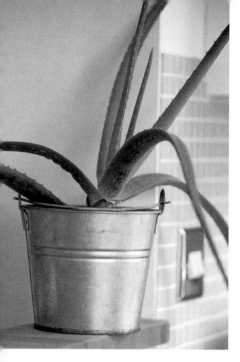

healing aloe

We probably all know aloe as a summer necessity for relieving sunburn, but with all of the nutrients it contains, it is no surprise that this super-plant offers many physical and mental-health benefits as well. Aloe is one of the few vegetarian sources of vitamin B12, and also contains vitamins A, C, E, folic acid, and choline. Potassium, calcium, selenium, and iron are among the 20 minerals it contains plus it has 19 amino acids, eight of which are essential.

Stir two teaspoons of the gel into 1 cup (8 fl oz/225 ml) glass of water for a refreshing aloe juice, which is a great general tonic recommended as an aid to digestion, a stimulus for intestinal health, and a gentle colon cleanse; or you could dilute the gel in an organic juice if you prefer.

Taking aloe vera daily will do you the world of good, but even just a couple of times a week will be beneficial. It can also be imbibed neat and, if you don't have your own plant, the juice is easily found at any grocery store nowadays, ready-made.

grow your own aloe

Even in colder climes, aloe can be grown inside in a wide pot with good drainage if you can find a sunny spot for it. If you're lucky enough to live somewhere warmer, an aloe plant will thrive outside and may even grow to tree-like proportions. Aloe propagates through baby plants sprouting off the sides, which you can repot into little clay containers and give as gifts to share the healing energy.

weight-loss tea

There is no quick or easy way to lose weight—it takes time and consistency. However, there are plenty of things you can do on a daily basis to encourage weight loss and maintenance. Basil is not usually found in common weight-loss teas but often weight gain can be due to over-toxicity in the body, especially the liver. Basil promotes detoxification of the liver, functions as an adaptogen in the body, and is anti-inflammatory. Green tea is rich in antioxidants, stabilizes blood sugar levels, and is rich in EGCG (epigallocatechin gallate—a polyphenol found in tea), which helps to combat obesity. Combined with lemon, ginger, and raw honey, this metabolism-boosting beverage can be enjoyed daily.

4–5 cups (950 ml–1.2 liters) water
1 teaspoon chopped fresh basil or ½–1 teaspoon dried basil
2 teaspoons green tea leaves
1-inch (2.5-cm) piece of fresh ginger, peeled and chopped
juice of 1 lemon
½ teaspoon raw honey

Serves 4

Put the water in a saucepan and bring to the boil. Add all the remaining ingredients except the honey, cover, and let boil for 5 minutes. Using a strainer or cheesecloth (muslin), strain the tea and pour into a thermos. Once the tea has cooled to a warm temperature, add the raw honey. Drink the tea throughout the day.

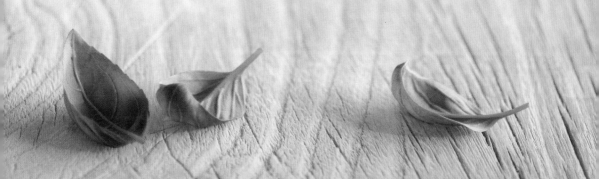

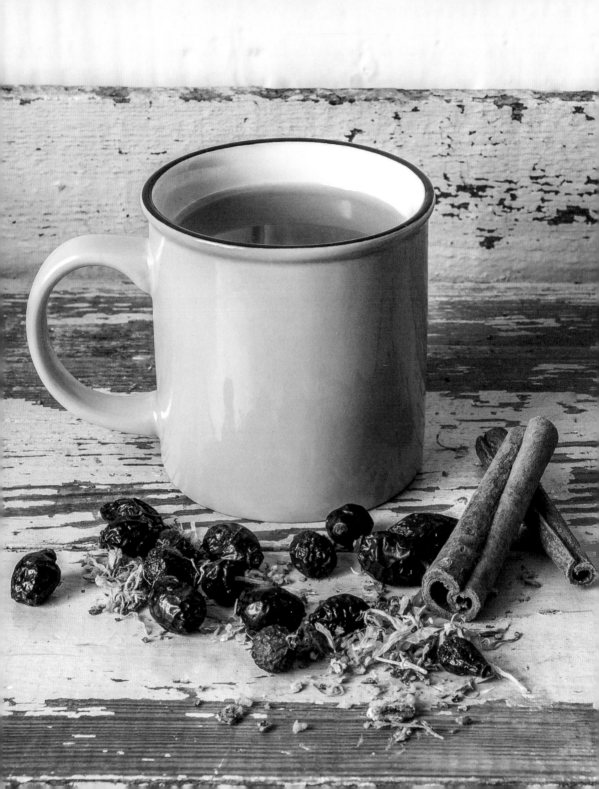

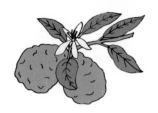

chapter 3

enhancing mental well-being

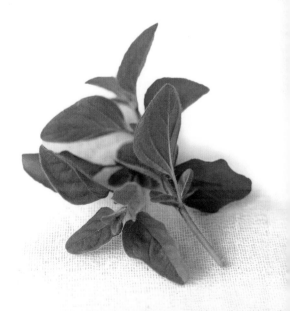

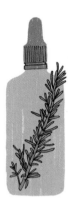

essential oil magic

Blending essential oils is both an art and a science. Combining these herbal oils can take their individual properties to the next level, interacting together to perform curative miracles.

A great blend involves combining notes—typically a top, middle, and base, though some blends don't require a base—to create a balanced and effective aroma. The top note is the first scent impression, which gives way to the middle note—the star of the show. The base note gives the blend its staying power and usually comes to the forefront much later. The aim in blending these three notes is to create a ratio that results in a harmonious cocktail that works (olfactorily or topically, depending on the blend) to address specific moods or ailments. A good rule of thumb is to use approximately 30 percent top note, 50 percent middle, and 20 percent base. If the blend doesn't require a base note, round it up to about 40 percent top and 60 percent middle. Always use the highest-quality organic essential oils (see Resources, page 140) for the best outcomes. Consult your local herbal apothecary and look for brands that have had GC/MS testing as that is known as the gold standard test for essential oils. I keep a stock of ½-ounce (15ml) dark-colored vials with stopper lids and blank labels for when aromatherapy needs arise.

For the following blends, carefully pour the oils into a vial and shake gently to blend. You can rub this on pulse points or use a diffuser. These are quite popular. If you are using a diffuser, no carrier oil is needed. I use the simplest and most old-fashioned kind of diffuser, which is a clay ring you can put at the base of a light bulb in a lamp. The warmth of the bulb slowly fills the space with the desired scent and effect. If you plan to use your blend on pulse points, you will need a carrier oil (see page 12). Always do a skin test first to avoid any potential irritation.

jubilance

The sweet scent of this blend makes you feel warm and fuzzy—euphoric, even.
* 1 drop each of top notes: bergamot, lemon, neroli
* 1 drop each of middle notes: ylang ylang, jasmine, Roman chamomile, geranium, rose
* 1 tablespoon of a carrier oil, ideally jojoba or apricot

quietude

If you need a moment of peace, try this citrus-floral blend.
* 3 drops of top note: orange
* 5 drops of middle note: ylang ylang
* 2 drops of base note: patchouli
* 1 teaspoon carrier oil, ideally sesame or jojoba

bright mind

Clear the mind and gain a keen sense of alertness with this bright, sunny blend.
* 1 drop each of top notes: rosemary, peppermint, bergamot, lemon
* 1 drop each of middle notes: mint, geranium, ylang ylang, jasmine, Roman chamomile
* 1 teaspoon carrier oil, ideally almond or grapeseed

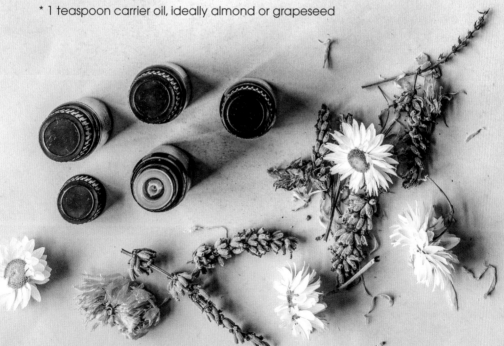

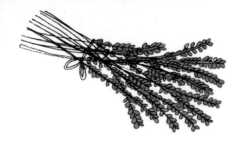

natural remedy blends

Both of the recipes here offer an excellent way to refresh and create personal space after a hectic week.

recipe 1

2 drops cedar essential oil

2 drops sandalwood essential oil

2 drops amber essential oil

2 drops lavender essential oil

4 drops carrier oil, such as sesame or jojoba

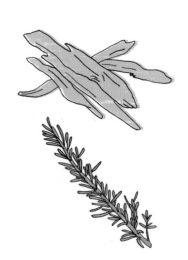

recipe 2

2 drops rosemary essential oil

3 drops bergamot essential oil

2 drops jasmine essential oil

3 drops lavender essential oil

6 drops carrier oil of your choice

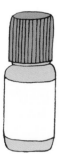

Blend the essential oils and carrier oil in a small ceramic or glass bowl. Gently rub one drop of Natural Remedy Potion on each pulse point: both wrists, behind your ear lobes, on the base of your neck, and behind your knees. As the oil surrounds you with its warm scent, you will be filled with a quiet strength.

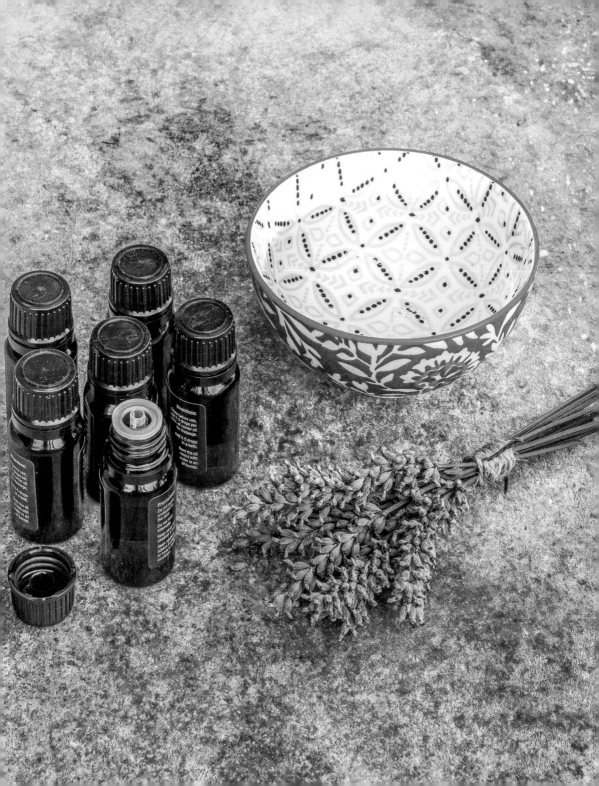

calm emotion potion

Why does every day seem to be as long as a week nowadays? Unplugging from cable news and constant social media feeds will help, as will this time-tested healing potion.

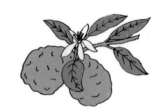

2 drops bergamot essential oil

2 drops vanilla essential oil

1 drop amber essential oil

2 drops lavender essential oil

4 drops carrier oil, ideally apricot or sesame

Mix all the oils together in a small ceramic or glass bowl. Gently rub one drop of Calm Emotion Potion on each pulse point: on both wrists, behind your ear lobes, on the base of your neck, and behind your knees. Close your eyes and breathe the sweetly serene scent in as you stand barefoot for 5 full minutes. If you need more time to restore yourself and regain your calm, continue your mindful breathing and contemplation. As the oil surrounds you with its warm scent, you will be filled with a quiet strength.

lemon and lavender lift blend

This is a miracle mix of oils that you should massage into your body for both stress relief and a moisturizer.

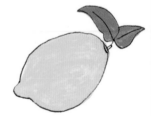

4 drops lavender oil

2 drops lemon oil

4 drops clary sage

5 teaspoons carrier oil, such as sesame

Put all the ingredients in a small, dark-colored dropper bottle and shake to mix. Keep this blend handy!

relaxation massage oil blend

Sandalwood, lavender, and clary sage create a deeply soothing blend with a sensuous scent. It is both restful and stimulating —the perfect combination.

- 6 drops sandalwood essential oil
- 6 drops lavender essential oil
- 6 drops clary sage essential oil
- ½ cup (120 ml) jojoba or almond carrier oil
- 1 cup (240 ml) warm water

Put the essential oils and carrier oil into a dark-colored, sealable bottle with a dropper cap. Carefully cap the bottle and gently shake until the oils have blended together. Store the bottle in a dark cupboard. Before using it on yourself or a loved one, shake well. You can warm it by putting the sealed bottle in a cup of warm water and let it sit there for 4 minutes. Many masseuses pour the oil into their palm and let their own body heat warm it. Either way adds to the relaxation factor.

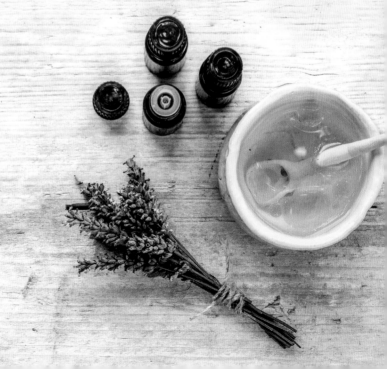

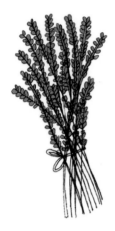

pulse-point lotion

Keep this homemade helpmate in your desk drawer where you can access it any time you need it. The lavender essential oil brings deeply tranquil feelings and vanilla is very comforting so this combination is ideal for a sense of zen positivity. In a mere ten minutes, you can whip up a spa retreat in lotion form.

½ cup (4 fl oz/125 ml) almond carrier oil

⅓ cup (2½ fl oz/75 ml) coconut oil

¼ cup (2 oz/60 g) shea butter

2 tablespoons beeswax

1 teaspoon each lavender essential oil and vanilla essential oil

Combine the almond and coconut oils, shea butter, and beeswax and heat gently in a double boiler. As the water heats, the ingredients will start to melt. Stir intermittently with a wooden spoon to blend. Once the mixture is melted, turn off the heat and remove from the stove. Once it has cooled for 5 minutes, gently fold in the essential oils so the batch is thoroughly infused. Pour into a sealable tin or heat-proof glass jar and seal.

The lavender essential oil brings deeply tranquil feelings and vanilla is very comforting so this combination is ideal for a sense of zen positivity. In addition to using the lotion on your hands, put a tiny bit on your fingertips and apply to your pulse points, such as your temples, wrists, over your heart, and at the base of your throat. Close your eyes and breathe in the delightful and relaxing scent and reclaim your zen.

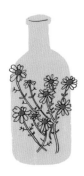

aromatherapy for anxiety

Welcome the scent of serenity into your daily life with these essential oils.

ROSE essential oil is extracted from the flowers' petals and has an exquisite perfume. Rose is highly prized for how it relaxes you and also stimulates the senses and memory.

LAVENDER is one of the most beloved of all aromatherapy oils and not just for the singular scent. It has been proven to relieve tension by the reaction of the limbic system in the brain that controls our emotions.

JASMINE essential oil has an arresting floral scent, which can encourage an increased sense of well-being. Jasmine calms the nervous system without causing sleepiness.

VETIVER oil is derived from the vetiver plant, a grassy native of India. It has a sweet, earthy scent and is used to attain a meditative state. It is a marvelous anti-anxiety remedy.

BASIL essential oil comes from the same herb that you use in cooking. In aromatherapy, it's used to help calm the mind and alleviate stress.

CLARY SAGE is a woody essential oil, valued for its anti-depressant qualities. It has been proven to reduce the body's production of cortisol, known as the stress hormone.

BERGAMOT, which comes from bergamot oranges, has a revitalizing citrusy scent. It is beloved for the way it can uplift and improve your mood.

YLANG YLANG, extracted from the flower of the tropical cananga tree, is highly floral and a great relaxant, also proven in scientific tests to lower tension, reduce blood pressure and even heart rate.

CHAMOMILE is pretty well-known for its relaxing and sedating properties and its appealing scent. Chamomile can help to overcome sleep disruptions and bring about a good, deep rest.

FRANKINCENSE oil, which is made from a tree resin, is cherished for its sweetly musky aroma, used to create a meditative state and ease anxiety.

LEMON BALM has a bracing and uplifting scent, which is very soothing and restorative and can also be a sleep aid.

VALERIAN has been used since ancient times to promote sleep and calm nerves. It can have a mild sedative effect on the body.

PATCHOULI has a musky, woodsy scent and is used in ayurvedic medicine to relieve anxiety, stress, and depression.

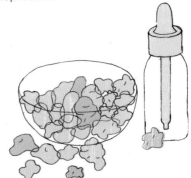

orange and spice blend

This can be used as a massage oil which is gently applied to pulse points. As a bonus, it repels bugs and can be great to use on a hiking or camping trip.

- 4 teaspoons apricot or jojoba carrier oil
- 4 drops cinnamon leaf essential oil
- 6 drops orange (neroli) essential oil

Pour these oils into a small, dark-colored dropper bottle. Shake gently and store in a dark cupboard for when you or your loved ones need perking up. Gently massaging the pressure points on your body is both pleasant and very therapeutic. This practice relieves pain, increases circulation, and perks up your personal energy. There are many pressure points to be found in soft tissue near bundles of nerves and joints. All should be kneaded tenderly.

bath sprinkle for peace

This homemade bath mix will create a peaceful scent while you bathe.

- 10 rose petals
- 5 sprigs lavender
- cheesecloth (muslin)

Crush the rose petals and lavender a little, then place in the middle of the cheesecloth (muslin) and tie the ends together to make a ball. Drop into a warm running bath.

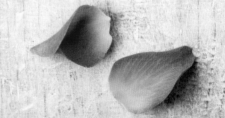

salt scrub to relax and aid sleep

This bath soak is marvelous for aromatic relaxation! The blend swiftly delivers serenity and a combination of full relaxation and heightened awareness. Magnesium flakes are easily available from health-food stores and pharmacies. The magnesium actually slows the production of the stress hormone in your body and aids sleep, as well as being marvelous for your skin.

handful of fresh mint leaves

½ cup (3½ oz/100 g) Epsom salts

½ cup (3½ oz/100 g) Himalayan pink salt

1 cup (7 oz/200 g) magnesium flakes

1 tablespoon Roman chamomile essential oil

12 drops lavender essential oil

4 drops neroli essential oil

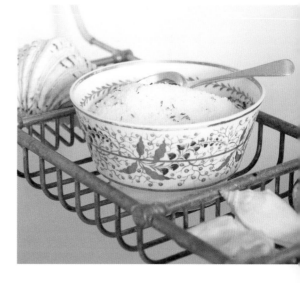

While you run a hot bath, crush the mint leaves in your hand and toss them directly into the hot water pouring from the faucet (tap). Now place all the salts in a metal bowl and gently fold in the magnesium flakes. Lastly, add the essential oils and stir lightly. Now pour half of the mixture under the faucet and when the bath is ready, disrobe and step in. Sit back and enjoy the delightful scent of the fresh mint and aromatherapy salts and oils. After a few minutes, take a loofah or a rough washcloth and use the remaining mix to scrub your skin. Afterward, sit for a spell and enjoy the stimulating sensations.

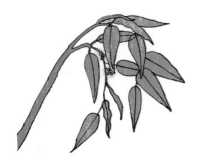

waters of wellness

For thousands of years, we humans have been "taking the waters" as a way to restore, and also heal illness. A bath that will simultaneously relax and stimulate you is a rare and wonderful thing.

4 cups (720 g) of Epsom salts
½ cup (120 ml) almond oil
6 drops comfrey essential oil
4 drops eucalyptus essential oil
4 drops rosemary essential oil
6 drops bergamot essential oil

Pour the salts into a large glass bowl and fold in the carrier oil. Now add in the essential oils, stirring after each is added. Continue to blend the mixture until it is moistened thoroughly. You can add more almond oil if necessary.

When your bathtub is one-quarter full, add one-quarter of the salt mixture under the faucet (tap). Breathe in deeply ten times, inhaling and exhaling fully.

When the tub is full, step inside and exercise your breath ten more times. Use the rest of the salts to scrub your body, carefully avoiding your eye area. Rest and rejuvenate as long as you like while visualizing your renewed health and vigor.

classic essential oils

Here are some healing solutions with common essential oils.

BERGAMOT: Calms anxiety and stimulates the mind.

YLANG YLANG Can help combat hypertension.

ROSEMARY: Kindles the memory and helps with perspiration.

LAVENDER: Can summon an instant sense of serenity by warming one drop between the palms of your hands.

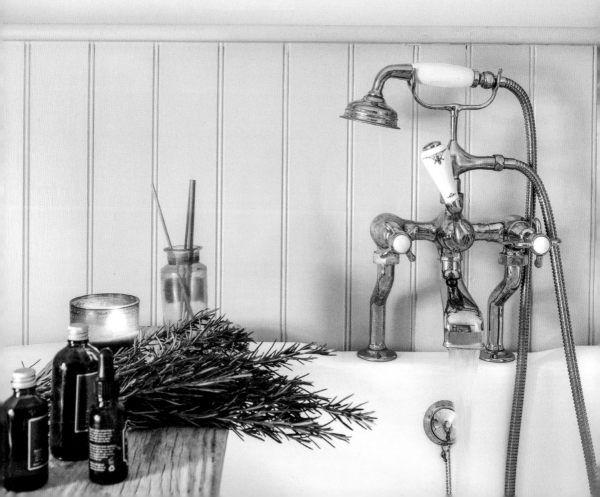

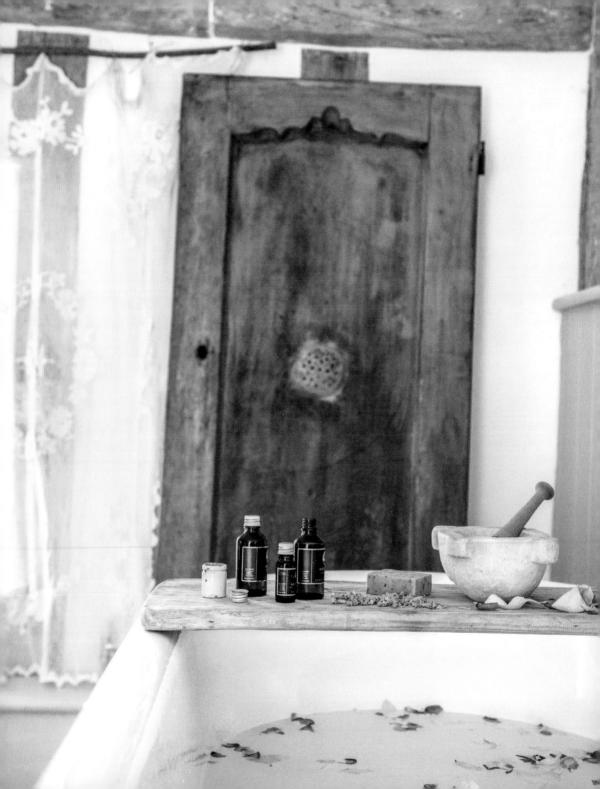

sensual soak

Sandalwood, amber, and vetiver are all rich, earthy scents that combine well together.

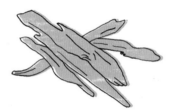

5 drops sandalwood essential oil

5 drops amber essential oil

2 drops vetiver essential oil

½ cup (90 g) Epsom salts

½ cup (70 g) baking soda

Combine the essential oils with the Epsom salts and stir in the baking soda. Mix well to create a richly scented paste. You can use a couple of different ways: either slather it onto yourself and shower off with a loofah and thick washcloth or, and this is my favorite way to soak up this earthly pleasure, roll it into a ball after you mix it and place under the faucet (tap) as you are running a hot bath. The entire room will smell like paradise. Soak it all in, lie back, and enjoy this fully. If you want to keep this for the future or give as a thoughtful gift, you can store in a lidded container or roll into bath bombs and let them dry on wax paper or paper towels. This recipe can make three palm-size bath bombs.

revitalizing herb tea

Prepare this tea as a pick-me-up and to balance your emotions.

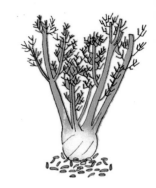

> 2 parts peppermint
> 1 part chamomile
> 1 part fennel

You can make a whole bag of the mixture and then brew a cup whenever you feel the need.

lavender and chamomile tranquility tonic

When we are fatigued, feelings of gloom can arise. This herbal healer can fend off the bad feelings and perk you right up. Herbal tonics, which are concentrated reductions of the herbs, last longer and provide a higher dose of the herb than teas or tisanes.

> 1½ cups (3 oz/80 g) dried lavender
> 1½ cups (3 oz/80 g) dried chamomile
> 1 cup (8 fl oz/225 ml) clear alcohol, such as vodka
> 2 cups (16 fl oz/450 ml) distilled water

Place the dried herbs into a clear 1-quart (1-liter) jar. Pour in the alcohol. Add in the distilled water, put on the lid securely, and shake for a few minutes until it seems well mixed. Store in a dark cupboard for 30 days, shaking once a day. Then strain through a 6-in. (15-cm) square of cheesecloth (muslin) into a dark glass storage jar and screw the lid on tightly. The lavender and chamomile leavings will make lovely compost for your garden and the liquid tonic will soon prove itself indispensable in your household.

quiet mind tea

If you ever feel overwhelmed and stressed out, it's a signal to your body to carve out some time for self-love. Taking a break from your everyday tasks to relax and quiet the mind is important. The tea's combination of four herbs works on the nervous system to calm feelings of being on edge and will instantly send you into a blissful state of relaxation. Brahmi is considered a nervine tonic due to its ability to intensely calm the nervous system and boost memory. Chamomile and lavender are anti-inflammatory and they bring a sense of peace and clarity to the body and mind. Valerian root works wonders for people suffering from anxiety, insomnia, chronic stress, and severe muscle cramps.

1 tablespoon dried brahmi leaf
1 tablespoon dried lavender flowers
1 tablespoon dried chamomile flowers
½ tablespoon dried valerian root
2 cups (475 ml) boiled water
raw honey, to taste

Serves 2

Put the herbs and boiled water in a bowl and let the mixture steep for 5 minutes. (If you oversteep the herbs, this tea will become very bitter and won't be as pleasant to drink.) Using a strainer or cheesecloth (muslin), strain the tea and pour into a thermos. Once the tea has cooled to a warm temperature, add the raw honey and enjoy!

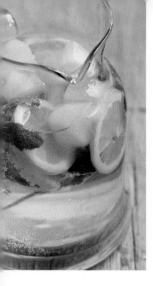

meadowsweet and apple mint calmer

Apple mint was used by monks in the Middle Ages to treat epilepsy—they believed it calmed the brain. This mint has a delicate sweet aroma of spearmint and apple, and is actually considered superior in taste to spearmint but lets itself down with its hairy leaves. We don't worry about that here—we embrace its fuzziness.

1 large handful apple mint leaves, stalks removed

2 large lemons, sliced into thin wheels

5 oz (150 ml) freshly squeezed lemon juice

7 oz (200 ml) Meadowsweet Syrup (see opposite) or store-bought elderflower cordial

3 cups (750 ml) organic cloudy apple juice

3 cups (750 ml) soda water

apple mint sprigs

elderflower/meadowsweet blossoms

Serves 6 (approximately 1 quart/1 liter)

Smack the mint leaves between your hands to release the essential oils, gently tear them, and drop into the pitcher. Add the lemon wheels, crushing them lightly to release some of their juice. Add the lemon juice, the Meadowsweet Syrup or elderflower cordial, and apple juice. Give it a good stir and place the pitcher in the refrigerator for at least an hour to chill properly and allow the flavors to marry.

When you are ready to serve, fill 6 glasses with ice. Fill each one two-thirds of the way up with the mix and top with soda water. Garnish with elderflower blossoms or meadowsweet blossoms (whichever are in season) and fresh apple mint sprigs.

meadowsweet syrup

15 heads of meadowsweet blossoms, fully opened

4 cups (1 liter) water

5 cups (1 kg) superfine (caster) sugar

zest and juice of 1 unwaxed, organic lemon

Makes approximately 1 quart (1 liter)

Strip the meadowsweet blossoms from the stems and stalks, and put to one side to give the wildlife plenty of time to evacuate.

Make a simple syrup by heating the sugar and water in a nonreactive pan over a low heat, stirring to dissolve the sugar. Once it reaches boiling point, remove the pan from the heat. Add the lemon zest and flowers. Submerge the flowers in the syrup, cover, and leave overnight or up to 12 hours, to infuse.

Add the lemon juice, stir, then strain into a wide-mouthed pitcher to remove the flowers and lemon zest. Reheat the syrup gently in a clean nonreactive pan and funnel into a sterilized presentation bottle(s) (see page 17) while still piping hot. Seal the bottle. Store somewhere cool and dark. Once opened, keep in the refrigerator for 2 to 3 months.

marvelous meadowsweet

There are records of meadowsweet being used medicinally since the 14th century. It is used for maintaining healthy sinuses and treating sinusitis, influenza, diabetes, and rheumatism. It's a cooling, aromatic, and astringent herb, famous for relieving pain—it contains salicylic acid, the active ingredient in aspirin. Its glorious floral scent makes it a favorite perfume ingredient. If that's not impressive enough, it's also been shown to have powerful antimicrobial benefits and be good at treating an acidic stomach and diarrhea.

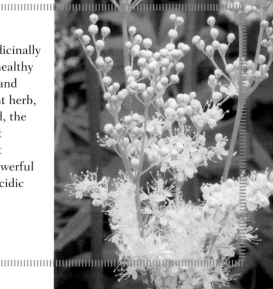

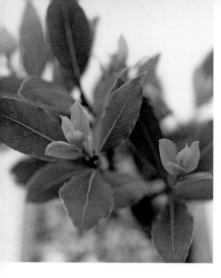

bay leaf balm to de-stress

Bay leaf balm will have a wonderfully calming effect anytime you use it and can be rubbed on your temples when you need to de-stress.

Any body oil or herbal oil can be turned into a salve with the addition of wax, and are simple to make. Balms are simply salves with the addition of essential oils.

If you have a bay laurel tree, pick some fresh leaves. You can also go to your spice rack and take three leaves from the jar and grind them in your mortar and pestle until broken up into fine, little pieces. Set aside a fourth whole leaf.

The ratio for a body salve is 3 oz (90 ml) coconut oil to 1 oz (30 ml) beeswax. Use a double boiler to heat the oil and wax until completely melted. Test the viscosity of your salve by pouring a dab onto a cold plate. If satisfied with the consistency, pour off into clean jars to cool. If you need to add more wax, now is the time to do it.

Add two drops of eucalyptus essential oil and two drops of lemon oil while the mix is still warm. Sprinkle in the finely crushed bay laurel, stir well, and seal to preserve the aroma.

To make the most of the balm, I recommend Sunday night soaks, where you slather on the balm before stepping into a hot bath. Take a washcloth and massage your skin, then lie back and relax for 20 minutes. When you drain the bathtub, your stress will also empty out, and you can start your week afresh, ready to handle anything that comes your way.

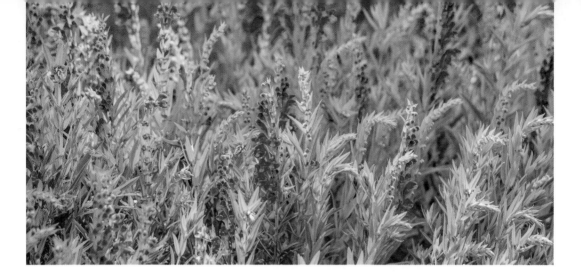

skullcap tincture for comfort and calm

This simple and easy recipe using the comforting skullcap herb makes a very fine tincture that has many medicinal uses. Your skullcap tincture will greatly alleviate anxiety and a downward spiral of moods. Even better, it comes in handy as a mouthwash and hair rinse and for baths, and even as a rub for achy joints and sore muscles.

¼ cup (½ oz/15 g) dried skullcap
2 cups (16 fl oz/450 ml) apple cider vinegar or 1 cup (8 fl oz/225 ml) vodka and 1 cup (8 fl oz/225 ml) water

Put the dried skullcap in a 1-quart (32-fl oz/1-liter) canning jar and carefully pour in the vinegar or vodka and water. Stir well and seal. Place on a dark shelf and shake once a day. After a month, strain through a 6-in. (15-cm) square of cheesecloth (muslin).

Compost the herbal residue in your garden and store the tincture in a 6-fl oz (175-ml) colored and sealable glass jar. Your tincture will keep for a year but you'll probably use it up much sooner!

For a cup of skullcap tea, add one teaspoon of the tincture to a cup of hot water, add a teaspoon of honey, stir, and enjoy.

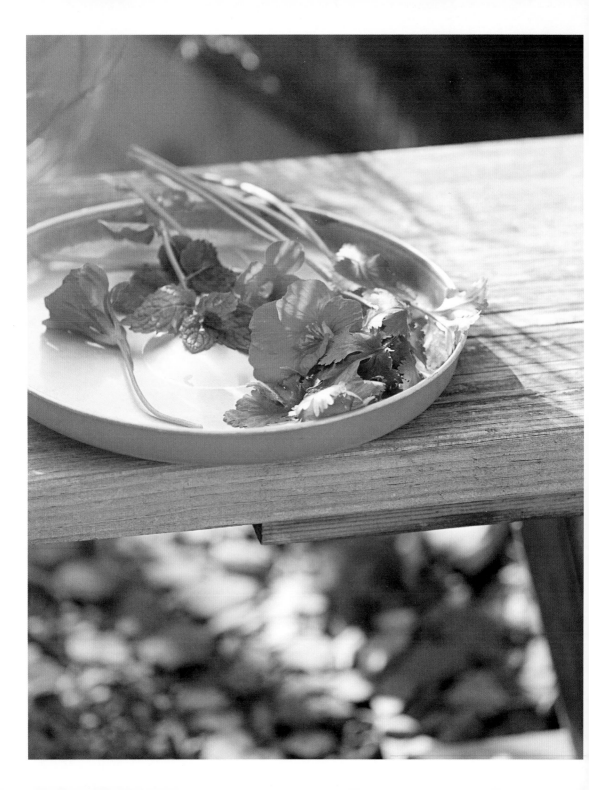

floral essence energies

Many of our favorite flowers have distinctive healing energies that can be captured in water. A key difference between flower essences and essential oils is that flower essences minister to the emotional body while essential oils treat the physical body.

Floral essences are also different from essential oils in that they do not carry the scent of the flower. It takes a few flowers to make an essence whereas essential oils rely on a significant amount of the plant.

Flower essences are typically ingested directly via the mouth or by way of adding a few drops to a glass of water. They can also be dropped onto linens, such as your pillowcase, or into your bath and can be applied directly to the pulse points (temples and wrists). I suggest using no more than two different floral waters at any given time for full effect.

Vials of a multitude of flower essences are available at grocers, pharmacies, and new-age shops. Bach Flower Remedies are doubtless the most popular and have a recommended dosage of three to four drops taken via the bottle dropper under the tongue two to four times a day. However, you can also make your own.

make your own flower essences

To make your own flower essences at home, start by making a mother tincture—the most concentrated form of the essence—which can then be used to make stock bottles. The stock bottles are used to make dosage bottles for the most diluted form of the essence, which is the one you actually take.

handful of freshly picked flowers specific to the malady being treated (see page 87)

6 pints (2.8 liters) fresh pure water or distilled water

organic brandy or vodka, at least 40 percent proof

Ideally, begin early in the morning, picking your chosen flowers (all of the same species) by 9 a.m. at the latest. This leaves you with three hours of sunlight before the noon hour, after which the sunlight is less effective, even draining.

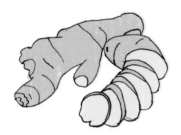

Put the water in a large glass mixing bowl. To avoid touching the flowers, use tweezers or chopsticks to place them carefully on the surface of the water, until the surface is covered. Leave the bowl in the sun for three to four hours, or until the flowers begin to fade.

Now, delicately remove the flowers, being careful not to touch the water. Strain the flower essence water through cheesecloth (muslin) into a large pitcher (jug). Half-fill a green or blue 8-fl oz (225-ml) sealable glass bottle with the flower essence water, and top up with the brandy or vodka (this will extend the shelf life of your flower water to three months if stored in a cool, dark cupboard). This is your mother tincture. Label it with the date and the name of the flower. Use any remaining essence water to water the flowers you've been working with.

TO MAKE A STOCK BOTTLE from your mother tincture, fill a 1-fl oz (30-ml) dropper bottle three-quarters full of brandy, top up with spring water, then add three drops of the mother tincture. This will last at least three months and enable you to make lots of dosage bottles.

TO MAKE A DOSAGE BOTTLE for any flower essence, just add two or three drops from the stock bottle to another 1-fl oz (30-ml) dropper bottle one-quarter full of brandy and three-quarters full of distilled water. Any time you need some of this gentle medicine, place 4 drops from the dosage bottle under your tongue or add it to a glass of water. Take or sip four times a day, or as often as you feel the need. You can't overdose on flower remedies, but you will find that more frequent, rather than larger, doses are much more effective.

flower essence remedies

One drop from a dosage bottle of flower essence mixed with 1 oz. (30 ml) distilled water can be used to remedy the following emotional conditions:

ADDICTION: agrimony, skullcap

ANGER: blue flag, chamomile, nettle

ANXIETY: aspen, garlic, gentian, lemon balm, nasturtium, periwinkle, rosemary, white chestnut

BEREAVEMENT: honeysuckle

DEPRESSION: black cohosh, borage, chamomile, geranium, larch, lavender, mustard, sunflower, yerba santa

EXHAUSTION: aloe, olive, sweet chestnut, yarrow

FEAR: basil, datura, ginger, mallow, peony, poppy, water lily

FOCUS AND CLARITY: lemon blossom

HEARTBREAK: borage, hawthorn, heartsease

LETHARGY: aloe, peppermint, thyme

SPIRITUAL BLOCKS: ginseng, lady's slipper, oak

STRESS: dill, echinacea, grape hyacinth, lemon balm, mistletoe, thyme

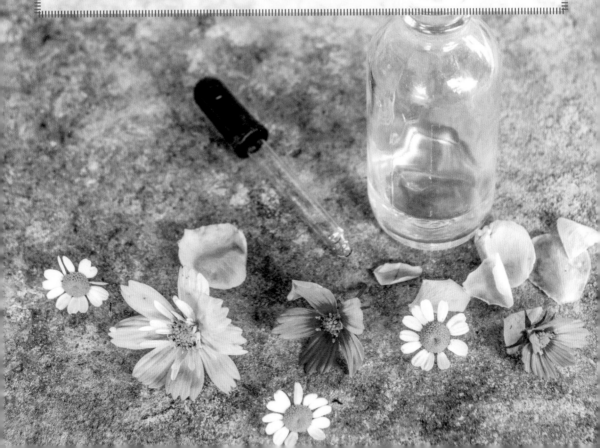

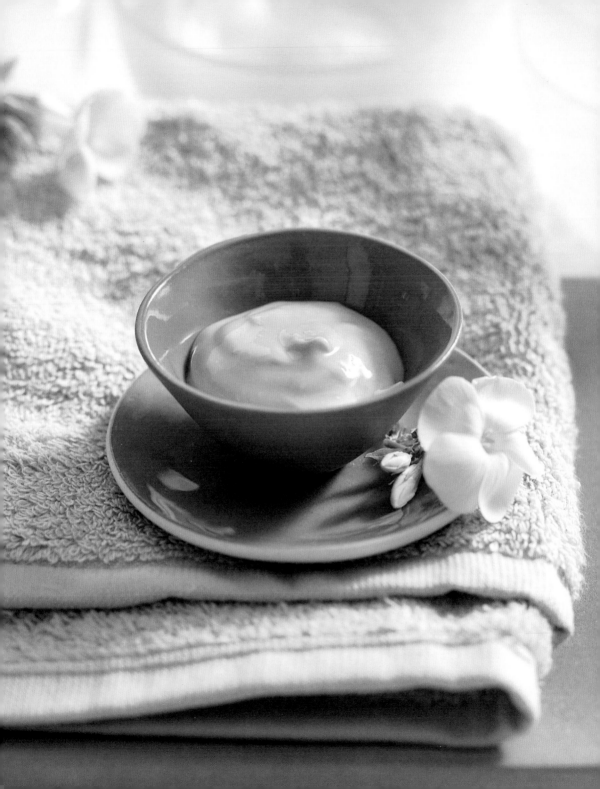

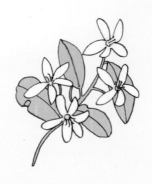

chapter 4

beauty solutions

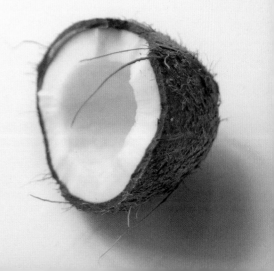

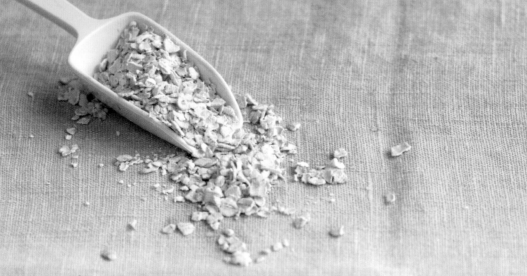

chamomile face mask

Warm oatmeal and chamomile tea conjure up a soothing feeling just at the thought of them—and they can also be an important part of your beauty regime.

up to 1 cup (225 ml) chamomile tea, steeped for a half hour

1 tablespoon honey

1 teaspoon baking soda (bicarbonate of soda)

½ cup (50 g) old-fashioned oats, ideally steel cut, crushed using a fork or ricer

2 tablespoon brown sugar

Put ½ cup (110 ml) chamomile tea in a small bowl and add the honey, baking soda (bicarbonate of soda), and oats. Add 2 tablespoons more tea to create an oaty paste. Set aside for 5 minutes. If the mixture is too dry, you can get the desired texture by adding a little more tea. Add the sugar and mix well.

Apply the face mask to clean, damp skin. Allow it to dry for 10 minutes, then rinse off thoroughly and massage your face gently with a natural moisturizer. Your skin will be miraculously smooth!

moringa mermaid mask

Moringa powder has antiseptic qualities. It fights and heals acne, reduces inflammation, is rich in vitamin A and amino acids that help produce collagen, and balances the skin's pH. This treatment's hydrating and collagen-building effects are great.

3 tablespoons water

juice of ½ lemon

½ teaspoon pearl powder

2 tablespoons raw honey

1½ tablespoons moringa powder

Makes enough for 1–2 uses

Cleanse and dry your skin. Mix all ingredients together in a small bowl until smooth. Apply the mask to your face with your fingertips or a facial mask brush, lightly massaging it into your skin. Leave the mask on for 15–20 minutes—lie down, walk around, or do whatever you like to do while the mask dries. Rinse off the mask with warm water. Any leftover mask will keep for up to 4 days in an airtight container in the refrigerator. When using the mask for the second time, you may need to add a little extra water to the mixture, one drop at a time, to loosen the mask to a useable consistency.

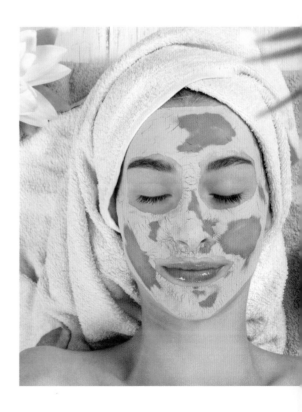

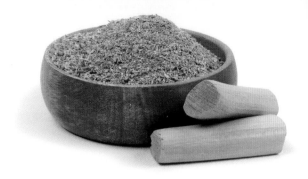

sandalwood shakti mask

Nutmeg and sandalwood have been used in Ayurvedic medicine for centuries to treat rashes, inflamed skin, cystic acne, and blemishes. This is the perfect face mask for anyone with inflamed skin. It's also ideal for anyone who is prone to acne due to its antibacterial cooling properties.

1 tablespoon ground nutmeg

4 tablespoons whole milk (raw if available)

2 tablespoons sandalwood powder

1 tablespoon raw honey

Makes enough for 1–2 uses

Cleanse and dry your skin. Mix all the ingredients together in a small bowl until smooth. Apply the mask to your face with your fingertips or a facial mask brush, lightly massaging it into your skin. Leave the mask on for 15–20 minutes, lying down with a towel beneath your head so the mask doesn't drip on anything (this mask tends to be a little watery). You may feel a tingling or stinging sensation while the mask is on. That is okay, the mask is working. Rinse off the mask with cool water. Any leftover mask will keep for up to 4 days in an airtight container in the refrigerator. When using the mask for the second time, you may need to add a little extra milk to the mixture, one drop at a time, to loosen the mask to a useable consistency.

blossoming beauty mask

If you have an oily and dull complexion with blackheads and clogged pores, use this exfoliating mask once or twice a week to brighten your complexion and tighten pores.

½ cup (100 g) goat milk yogurt (raw if available)

½ teaspoon rose water

1 tablespoon pink clay powder

1 tablespoon triphala powder (see page 26)

½ teaspoon raw honey

a spritz of Citrus-Rose Hydrosol (see page 97)

Makes enough for 1–2 uses

Cleanse and dry your skin. Mix all the ingredients together in a small bowl until smooth. Apply the mask to your face with your fingertips, lightly massaging it into your skin to give yourself a slight exfoliation. Leave the mask on for 15–20 minutes —lie down, walk around, or do whatever you like to do while the mask dries. Rinse off the mask with warm water. Mist your skin with the Citrus-Rose Hydrosol. Any leftover mask will keep for up to 4 days in an airtight container in the refrigerator. When using the mask for the second time, you may need to add a little extra yogurt to the mixture, one drop at a time, to loosen the mask to a useable consistency.

glowing goddess face oil

This face oil is suitable for all skin types. You can use it as a daily moisturizer, serum, or at any moment when you're in need of some self-love.

2 tablespoons jojoba oil

1 tablespoon sea buckthorn oil

1 tablespoon carrot seed oil

1 tablespoon tamanu oil

1 teaspoon rose hip oil

20–30 drops hyaluronic acid

2 drops of geranium essential oil

2 drops of frankincense essential oil

2 drops of lavender essential oil

2 drops of sandalwood essential oil

Makes about 4 fl oz (120 ml)

Mix all the ingredients together in a small bowl. Using a funnel, transfer the oil to a 4-fl-oz (120-ml) glass jar or bottle. Store in a cool, dark place. This oil will keep for up to 6 months. Massage your face daily with the oil to enhance your skin's radiance and keep it supple.

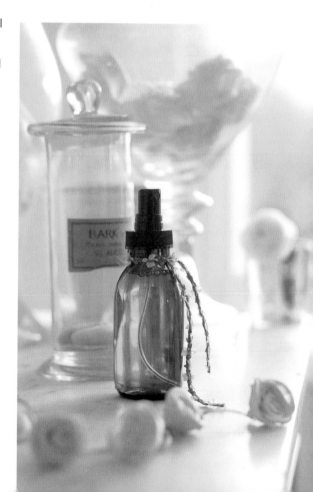

moringa morning matcha tonic

If you've never tried matcha tea, it's one of the most decadent and velvety smooth teas you'll ever taste. Matcha is rich in EGCG (see page 61), which is crucial for antiaging. You probably won't find moringa and matcha combined at your local tea or coffee shop, but this is an easy pick-me-up you can make at home. You don't need professional matcha tea equipment, just a small bowl and a whisk.

½ cup (120 ml) almond milk

1 teaspoon matcha green tea powder

¼ cup (60 ml) hot water

½ teaspoon moringa powder

½ teaspoon mucuna pruriens powder

raw honey or stevia, to taste

Serves 1

Heat the almond milk in a small saucepan over a medium-low heat for 3 minutes or until the milk slightly bubbles. Meanwhile, put the matcha in a small bowl and add the hot water. Whisk until the matcha has completely dissolved and become smooth. Transfer the almond milk to a food processor or blender, add the moringa and mucuna pruriens, and blend until smooth. Pour into a mug, top with the matcha, and stir together. Once the liquid has cooled to a warm temperature, add the honey or stevia.

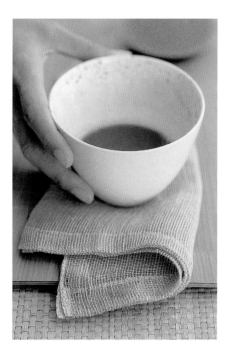

rose renewal spray

Use this spray to freshen your face in the morning or after being in a stuffy room.

10 fl oz (0.3 liters) water

2 tablespoons crushed rose petals

2 tablespoons rosemary

5 eucalyptus leaves

1 tablespoon vitamin C (you can get pure vitamin C—also called ascorbic acid—in pharmacies or health-food stores, but if you cannot obtain it, use a crushed vitamin C tablet)

Bring the water to a gentle simmer, then add the rose petals, rosemary, and eucalyptus. Do not boil! Leave simmering for 15 minutes. Cool to room temperature, then strain out the herbs and add the vitamin C. Pour into a dark spray bottle. It will keep for a couple of weeks if refrigerated.

You can also use this as a make-up remover if you double the quantity of water to dilute it.

apple skin toner

Apple cider vinegar (see page 49) will become one of your best-loved beauty fixes and a household mainstay. To make a skin-soothing facial toner, mix one part water and one part apple cider vinegar and wipe gently over a clean face using a cotton swab or soft clean cloth.

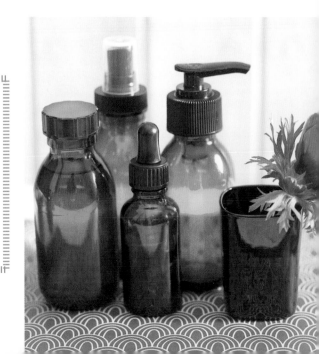

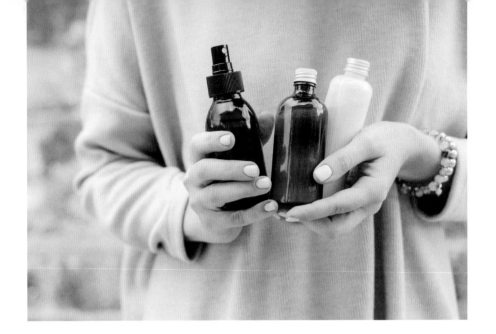

citrus-rose hydrosol

A hydrosol is simply a misting moisturizer. It is the perfect soothing pick-me-up for your skin, whether for first thing in the morning or when you're out and about.

1–4 mini rose quartz crystals

½ cup (120 ml) alkaline or purified water

2 drops of colloidal silver

1 teaspoon rose water

4 drops of citrus essential oil

Makes about 4 fl oz (125 ml)

Place the rose quartz crystals at the bottom of an empty 6-fl-oz (175-ml) spray bottle, then add the remaining ingredients. Shake to mix and it's ready to spray! This hydrosol should keep for up to 1 month, or even longer if you store it in the refrigerator.

beauty ambrosia tea

The word ambrosia means "immortality" in Greek. If you want clear, radiant, glowing skin, it must come from within—what we put on our skin is just an extra bonus. Hibiscus, rose, and calendula all help to remove excess heat from the blood, heal the heart, and tonify the skin.

3 tablespoons dried hibiscus flowers

2 tablespoons dried calendula flowers

2 tablespoons dried red or pink rose petals

2 cups (475 ml) boiled water

raw honey, to taste

Serves 2

Put the herbs and boiled water in a bowl and let the mixture steep for 1 hour or until the liquid is a vibrant red color. Using a strainer or cheesecloth (muslin), strain the tea and pour into a thermos. Once the tea has cooled to a warm temperature, add the raw honey. Enjoy the tea warm or at room temperature.

adaptogenic beauty milk

Use this powerful beauty milk daily to build your radiance from within and achieve glowing clear skin and radiant hair.

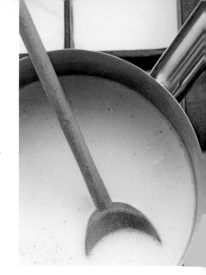

1½ cups (350 ml) water

½ cup (120 ml) almond milk

1 tablespoon pearl powder

1 tablespoon amalaki powder

½ tablespoon schizandra berry

1 teaspoon raw honey

Serves 1

Put the water and almond milk in a small saucepan and cook over a low heat for 3 minutes or until it comes to a low boil. Transfer the mixture to a food processor or blender, add all the remaining ingredients except the honey, and blend on high until the milk gets frothy. Once the liquid has cooled to a warm temperature, add the honey. Drink out of your favorite mug.

beautifying oil

Use as a massage oil or as a moisturizing oil for your hands.

10 drops citronella oil

10 drops geranium oil

20 drops orange oil

20 cumin seeds

3⅓ fl oz (100ml) almond oil

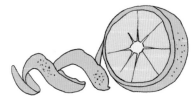

Combine the ingredients by adding the essential oils and cumin seeds slowly into the almond oil one by one.

saffron and lemon elixir

Saffron is widely used in Ayurvedic medicine for its ability to beautify the skin, boost moods, decrease feelings of depression, and combat PMS and infertility in both men and women.

½-inch (1-cm) piece of fresh ginger, peeled and grated
½ teaspoon saffron threads
juice of 1 lemon
2 tablespoons monk fruit sugar
4–5 cups (950 ml–1.2 liters) water

Serves 4

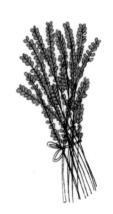

Put the ginger, saffron, lemon juice, and monk fruit sugar in a small saucepan over a low heat, then add the water and let the liquid come to the boil. Remove from the heat, cover, and let stand for 20 minutes. There's no need to strain this tea. Pour the liquid into a thermos and enjoy the tea hot or at room temperature. You can also freeze the tea in ice-cube trays and add the ice cubes to room-temperature water—the ice cubes make the water a beautiful color.

ageless skin potion

This oil takes excellent care of your skin..

¼ cup (60 ml) sweet almond oil (as a base)
2 drops chamomile oil
2 drops rosemary oil
2 drops lavender oil

Combine these oils in a sealable, dark bottle. Shake very thoroughly to mix. Clean your skin with warm water, then gently daub with the mixture.

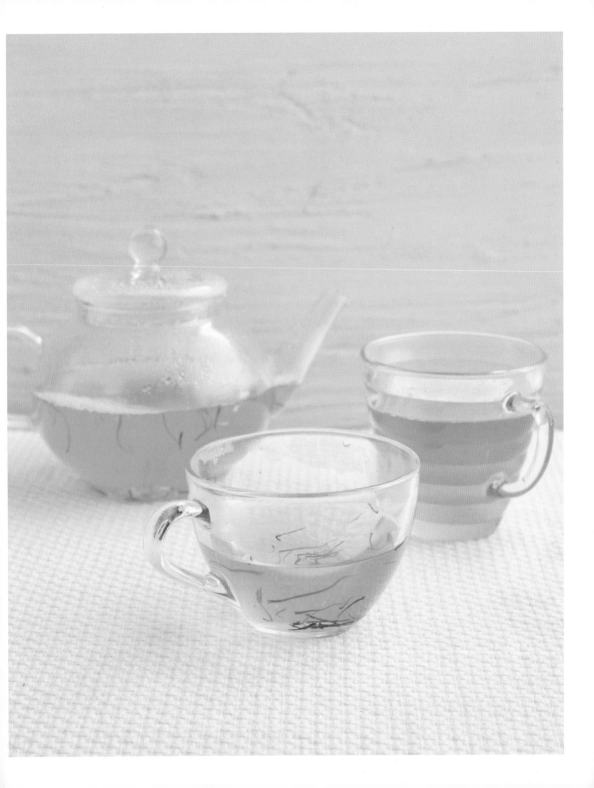

soothing self-massage

Massage has been shown to provide deep nourishing and cleansing effects on the entire bodily system.

This self-massage is done by massaging warm herbal oil onto the entire body before bathing. It helps to nourish the tissues of the body; stimulates the organs; increases circulation; slows down aging; brings longevity; softens, clears, and increases firmness of the skin; helps combat insomnia; detoxes the lymphatic system; and clears the channels of the body.

Opposite is an easy step-by-step guide to help you incorporate this ancient practice into your everyday self-care routine. The massage starts at the top of your head and works its way down the front and back of your body. You can oil just the top of your scalp or you may choose to oil your entire head, including your hair. Remember to always test oils on a small patch of your skin to ensure you are not allergic before you apply the oil all over your body.

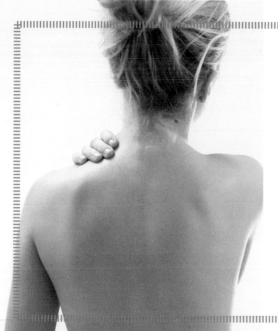

make your own self-massage oil

To enhance your massage, you can add essential oils (see page 64) to a carrier oil (see page 12). Add 10–20 drops of your preferred essential oil—you can mix different ones together if you like—to a 12-fl oz (350-ml) container of your carrier oil.

how to perform self-massage

1 Warm 4–8 fl oz (120–250 ml) massage oil in a heat-safe container, such as a ceramic, glass, or BPA-free plastic bowl, to a little warmer than body temperature. Either warm the oil in a double boiler/bain-marie on the stove to manage the temperature more efficiently, or heat the oil in the microwave in 30-second increments, testing the temperature as you go. To test the temperature of the oil, carefully apply a small spot of oil to your wrist to make sure it is not too hot.

2 Stand on an old towel in your bathroom—the towel will catch any excess oil so it doesn't stick to the floor.

3 Pour some oil into the palms of your hands, the more oil the better! Cover your entire body with the oil.

4 Using small circular strokes, massage the crown of your head. If you don't want oil in your hair, begin the massage at your ears. Avoid using the oil on your face, except for your ears and neck.

5 Using upward strokes and an open hand to create friction, massage the front and back of your neck.

6 Using a clockwise circular motion, massage around your breasts/chest.

7 Using a clockwise circular motion, massage your stomach/abdominal area. You really need to work in deep here. If you are pregnant, recovering from surgery, or have chronic pain in this area, consult a specialist before deeply massaging the area.

8 Using long up and down strokes, rub one of your arms to create friction and heat. Once you have created heat, massage the entire arm with a circular motion, starting at the bottom of the wrist and working upward toward the heart on the inside of the arm. Repeat on the other arm.

9 Add some extra oil to your hands and, without straining, reach around to your back and spine and gently massage with up and down strokes.

10 Vigorously massage up and down your legs up to create friction and heat. Focus on the top of one thigh and work your way down the leg, taking care to work your hands in a circular motion on the insides of your legs (this is a huge lymphatic part and many toxins build up in these areas). Repeat on the other leg.

11 Take some extra time to work the oil into your feet.

12 Once you've finished the massage, take a warm shower or bath for as long as feels comfortable. The idea is to open the pores to let the oil sink in deeper. Don't use soap to wash off the oil (it's not necessary). Towel dry after you shower or bathe. Take caution when stepping out of the bathtub or shower, as the floor may be slippery.

yummy spa scrubs

Gentle abrasives in the form of body scrubs exfoliate and stimulate the skin—the body's largest organ—while helping it to stay nourished and moisturized. Massaging yourself with these is also good for the lymphatic system. Here are four simple scrub combinations for you try. For each one, stir the ingredients together in a bowl until well mixed (you may need more or less oil than specified), then decant into glass jars. Rinse the bathtub or sink thoroughly after use to avoid stains or stickiness.

zesty lemon sugar scrub

- ½ cup (100 g) white sugar
- 2 tablespoons lemon juice
- 1 teaspoon lemon zest
- 1 tablespoon olive oil

coconut colada sugar scrub

- 1 cup (85 g) brown sugar
- 3 tablespoons melted coconut oil
- 1 teaspoon each ground cinnamon and ground cloves

morning brew coffee scrub

- ½ cup (85 g) coffee grounds
- ½ cup (100 g) fine sea salt
- 1-2 tablespoons almond oil

vanilla sugar scrub

- ¼ cup (45 g) brown sugar
- ¼ cup (45 g) white sugar
- ¼ cup (60 ml) organic olive oil
- 6-8 drops vanilla essential oil

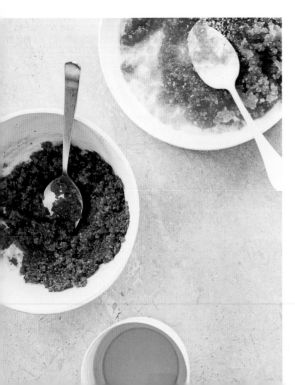

body purification bath scrub

Since the time of the ancients in the Mediterranean and Mesopotamia, salts of the sea combined with soothing oils have been used to purify the body by way of gentle, ritualized rubs. Dead Sea salts have long been a popular export and are readily available at most health food shops and spas. However, you can make your own salts, and not only control the quality and customize the scent, but save money, too.

3 cups (385g) Epsom salts
½ cup (120ml) sweet almond oil
1 tablespoon glycerin
4 drops ylang-ylang essential oil
2 drops jasmine essential oil

Mix well and store in a colored and well-capped glass bottle. Use these salts with a clean washcloth or new sponge and gently scrub your body while standing in the shower or bathtub. You will glow with health and inner peace.

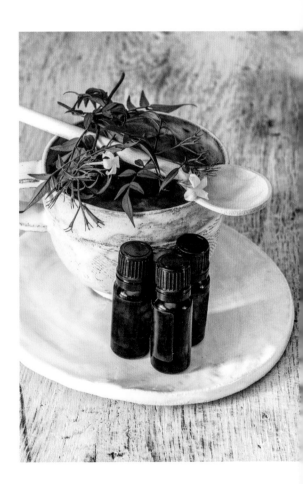

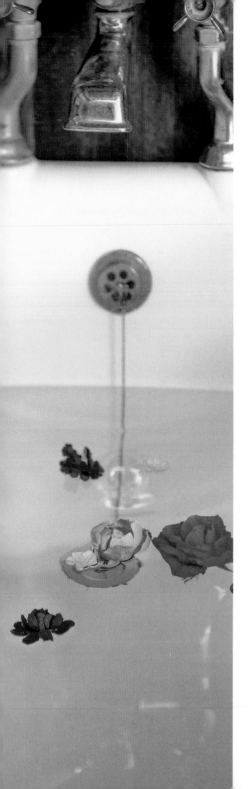

rose milk bath

You couldn't dream up a more luxurious bath for your skin than this concoction. The lactic acid in the milk helps to remove dead skin, while the rose oil calms and tones new skin.

1½ cups (190 g) milk powder (raw if available)
½ cup (130 g) Himalayan pink salt
1 handful dried or fresh rose petals
10 drops of rose essential oil

Makes enough for 1 use

Put all the ingredients except the rose petals in a bowl of warm water and stir until the milk powder and salt dissolve. Fill your bathtub with water, then add the milk and salt mixture and sprinkle in the rose petals. Soak in the bath for 20 minutes–1 hour.

detox bath

These invigorating bath salts help to draw toxins out of the body and soften the skin.

2 cups (450 g) Epsom salts
1 cup (225 g) baking soda (bicarbonate of soda)
10 drops of ginger essential oil
1 large lemon, washed and sliced

Makes enough for 1 use

Fill your bathtub with warm water and then add all the ingredients. Soak in the bath for 20 minutes–1 hour.

relaxing chamomile bath

Adaptogens (see pages 14-15) are an amazing additive for our daily lives—ashwagandha powder can help calm and relax nervousness and anxiety. Magnesium flakes are crucial for the remineralization of the body.

1 cup (225 g) magnesium flakes

10 drops of chamomile essential oil

½ cup (70 g) ashwagandha powder

1 handful fresh rose petals, lavender, chamomile, or other wild flowers (optional)

Makes enough for 1 use

Put all the ingredients except the fresh flowers, if using, in a bowl of warm water and stir until the magnesium flakes and ashwagandha powder dissolve. Fill your bathtub with water, then add the bath salts and sprinkle in the flowers, if using. Soak in the bath for 20 minutes–1 hour.

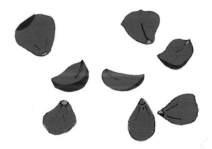

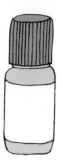

neroli and vanilla calming balm

This basic three-ingredient recipe takes all the fuss and muss away so you even enjoy the process of creating your own calming balm. The concoction will not only soothe and nourish the skin, but also it is very good for your soul. The fresh and lightly citrus scent of neroli in combination with vanilla is extremely comforting and also tremendously relaxing. The result is so pleasing that you may even consider using it as a perfume.

1 cup (8 oz/225 g) shea butter
½ cup (4 fl oz/125 ml) coconut oil
½ cup (4 fl oz/125 ml) almond oil
15 drops neroli essential oil
15 drops vanilla essential oil

Melt the shea butter with the coconut oil in the top of a double boiler. Remove from the heat and allow to cool for 30 minutes. Add in the almond oil (you can substitute olive oil, jojoba oil, or any liquid organic oil) and blend. When the mixture starts to solidify partially, add in 15 drops each of the essential oils. Stir in, and then whip the mixture to a butter-like consistency, which will take a few minutes only.

Store the balm in 4-fl oz (125-ml) clean, glass-lidded jars in a cool, dry cupboard. This balm also makes a thoughtful gift.

more mood-boosting balm blends

Try these alternative combinations for the balm recipe opposite and you will soon discover bliss in a bottle.

MELLOW ME: equal parts of chamomile and rose is a gentle, mellowing combination.

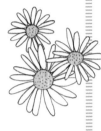

IN YOUR GROOVE: bergamot and basil will help you to get your groove back.

CHILL OUT: clary sage and ylang ylang pair up nicely to bring you peace of mind.

UNWIND YOUR MIND: jasmine and valerian will sweeten up your mood in a jiffy.

HAPPY HIPPIE: lavender and patchouli are a power duo for a quiet mind and upbeat thinking.

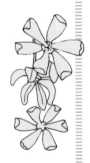

SWEET SERENITY: lemon balm and vetiver combine for real soothing and letting go of tension.

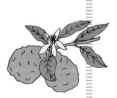

nourishing lip gloss

With this simple recipe, your lips will be soft, luscious, and super shiny.

2 oz (50 g) beeswax

2 oz (50 g) castor oil

beet juice

2 drops of any edible essential oil if desired, such as allspice, cinnamon, citronella, sage, lavender, peppermint, basil, clove, nutmeg, rosemary, or jasmine

catnip leaves

Melt the beeswax and add the castor oil. Add beet juice (how much will depend on how red you want your lip gloss to be—the more beet you add, the deeper the color). Then add the drops of essential oil to give the lip gloss flavor. Line a small jar with catnip leaves and pour in the mixture. Leave to cool, and it's ready to use!

raspberry lip balm

Once you have all the right ingredients it's very easy to make your own lip balm – and once you start, you'll never go back to the store-bought variety. Beeswax is the key ingredient; it's completely natural, it makes the lip balm stay hard, plus it's an excellent lip protector and moisturizer. There are also some extra moisturizing ingredients, in the form of vitamin E oil and jojoba oil, to take good care of your lovely lips. The raspberries give your lips a slight hint of pink the natural way.

1½ tablespoons freeze-dried raspberries

2 tablespoons pure jojoba oil

1½ teaspoons natural beeswax pellets (see note)

10 drops pure vitamin E oil

1 drop rose or lavender essential oil (optional)

Grind the freeze-dried raspberries in a coffee grinder or small food processor until very fine. Gently heat the jojoba oil and beeswax together in a double boiler (a small heatproof bowl set over a saucepan of simmering water), or in a microwave on its lowest setting for a few seconds. When melted, remove from the heat and add the vitamin E oil, raspberry powder and, if you wish, a drop of rose or lavender essential oil. Pour the mixture into a 1½-oz (45ml) jar with a lid and leave to set. It keeps for up to a month. The raspberry powder can feel a bit grainy on the lips, but rub your lips together and use it like an exfoliant, leaving your lips feeling super-soft.

Note: It is easier to buy beeswax in pellet form, as the blocks are difficult to cut for small quantities.

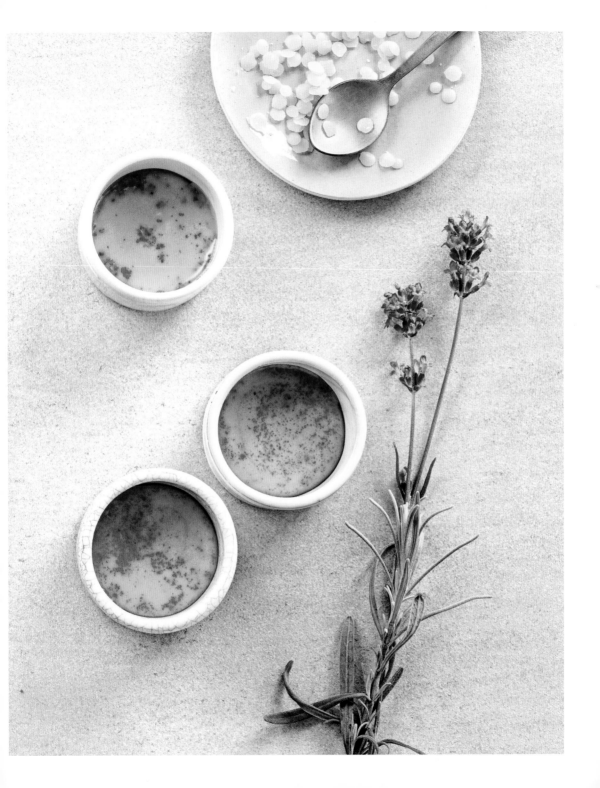

grapefruit and almond joy lotion

Once known as "the forbidden fruit of Barbados," grapefruit awakens the mind and body. Like many other citrus fruits, it is cheering to the mood and renowned for what it does for skin–it can even reduce cellulite. Almond is prized as an erotic massage oil. This mixture is a real treat: a creamy body lotion that glides on and does not feel heavy. A mixer is ideal for making it, but if you don't have one, use a hand whisk.

2 tablespoons raw shea butter (at room temperature)

½ cup (110 g) virgin coconut oil (which is solid at room temperature)

2 cups (450 ml) almond oil

2 tbsp grapefruit zest

2 teaspoons tapioca flour

Place the shea butter, coconut oil, almond oil, and grapefruit zest in the bowl of a mixer fitted with the whisk attachment. Mix on medium power for 30 seconds, then turn to high and mix for about 4 minutes, until it is light and fluffy. Scrape the sides of the bowl as needed to make sure everything is combined. Add the tapioca flour and mix for 1 minute. Transfer to a jar with a lid. The lotion will keep at room temperature for up to a month.

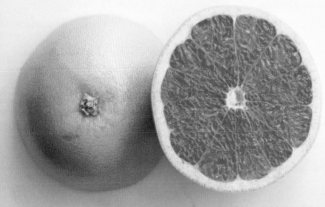

skin-nourishing body whip

Lather this decadent mixture all over your skin as you get into the bathtub, then ease down into the water and just soak. It is fabulously luxurious and will nourish your skin wonderfully.

    1 cup (220 g) virgin coconut oil (which is solid at room temperature)
    4 drops essential oil of your choice

Put the coconut oil in a medium-sized bowl. Using a hand mixer or an electric mixer with a whisk attachment, whip the oil until it reaches a soft consistency, like whipped cream. Add essential oil and whip to combine. Use every bit for your treatment; you deserve it.

mint miracle foot therapy

After a long day at the office, out hiking, or even dancing, your feet will be "dog tired." This pick-me-up will soon have you out and about again, feeling fresh and fabulous.

    handful of crushed mint leaves
    3 tablespoons solid coconut oil, warmed and softened
    1 teaspoon white vinegar or apple cider vinegar (see page 49)
    3 drops mint essential oil

Grind the mint leaves thoroughly into the coconut oil using a pestle and mortar. Transfer to a bowl, then stir in the vinegar and essential oil. Place the mix in the freezer for 5 minutes. Sit on the side of the bathtub and gently massage the mix into your feet, giving every toe and heel lots of loving attention. Take your time—your feet do a huge amount of work all day, every day. When you are satisfied, rinse your feet clean in the shower. Now, you deserve to put your feet up and just enjoy life for a while.

blissful massage bars

Massage bars should look, smell, and feel luxurious. Cocoa butter is beloved for its delicious chocolate scent, but you could also use sumptuous shea butter or mango butter. Use your favorite essential oil to create a scent you will love.

> 3 oz (80 g) beeswax
> ½ cup (120 ml) almond oil
> 3 oz (80 g) cocoa butter
> 1 teaspoon essential oil of your choice

Heat the beeswax, almond oil, and cocoa butter slowly a bain-marie or double boiler over a low heat until just melted. Remove from the heat and let cool slightly. Stir in the essential oil. Pour the mix into soap bar molds and let cool for about 2 hours, until hardened. Place in the freezer for a few minutes to make it easier to pop the bars out of the molds. To use, rub the massage bar onto the skin—the warmth of your body will immediately begin to melt the bar.

moisturizing coconut bath

Coconut milk creates a rich, moisturizing bath and leaves skin silky smooth. Ylang ylang is a heady, exotic scent that is lightened and heightened by the citrusy note of the orange.

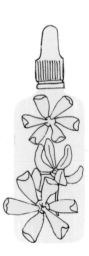

> 2 drops ylang ylang essential oil
> 3 drops orange essential oil
> 1 can (14 fl oz/400 ml) of coconut milk

Combine the essential oils with the coconut milk and add to a tubful of warm water.

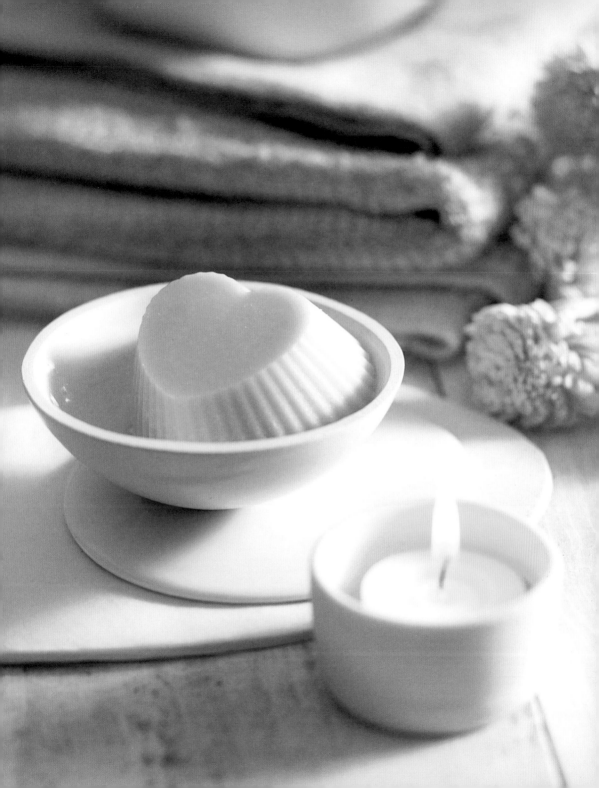

homemade haircare

The chemicals in haircare products can contribute to early hair loss, so detox your routine as much as possible. Instead of coating your head in chemical compounds such as sodium lauryl sulfate and artificial fragrances, which can be toxic, you can make your own products. In doing so, you will also avoid contributing to the problem of plastic waste.

baking soda shampoo

- 1 cup (225 ml) warm water
- 1 tablespoon baking soda (bicarbonate of soda)

Pour the water into a large bowl, add the baking soda (bicarbonate of soda), and stir well until it has dissolved. Now, pour over wet hair. Rub the mixture into your hair, paying special attention to massaging your scalp. If you tend to have oily hair, concentrate your efforts around the hairline and the crown of the head. If you have long hair, you can double the amounts. Rinse thoroughly and dry as normal.

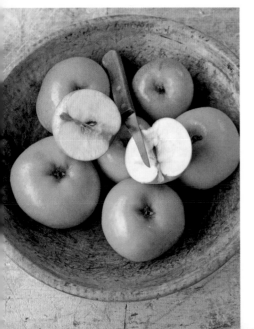

apple hair conditioner

1 cup (225 ml) warm water

2 tablespoons apple cider vinegar (see page 49)

Mix the water and vinegar in a bowl and pour over freshly shampooed hair. Gently massage into your hair and scalp and leave for a few moments before rinsing. After a couple of months of DIY hair love, your tresses will be shockingly shiny.

tonics and rinses

To improve the condition of your scalp and make your hair strong and shiny, experiment with the following herbal treatments.

BRIGHTENING FAIR HAIR: Chamomile water in the final rinse is good for fair hair—pour boiling water over fresh chamomile flowers, leave for an hour, and use when cooled.

ADDING SHINE TO DARK HAIR: Rosemary tea as a final rinse leaves dark hair shiny and glossy.

NETTLE SCALP TONIC: Not only do nettles have a good reputation for encouraging hair growth; they also eliminate dandruff. Boil a large rubber-gloved handful of nettles in water and simmer for 10 minutes, cool, and strain the liquid. Store it in the fridge and use when required.

HORSETAIL HAIR TONIC: A common and invasive weed, horsetail may be growing, uninvited, in your garden. Steep a bunch of horsetail in simmering water for 20 minutes. This decoction can be used as a tonic to strengthen your hair. After shampooing, rinse and pour a pitcherful of cooled horsetail water over your hair, wrap your head in a warm towel for 20 minutes, then rinse. The lotion can also be used as a nail strengthener.

PARSLEY SEED HAIR TONIC: Crush parsley seeds and steep them in water to make a hair rinse that will leave hair shiny and glossy. It is also said to eliminate head lice. Pour the rinse over your head and wrap in a towel for an hour. Do not rinse off, and allow hair to dry naturally.

MALT VINEGAR HAIR TONIC: To add a glowing shine to your hair, add half a cup of malt vinegar to the final rinse.

STRENGTHENING HAIR RINSE: For stronger hair, place 5 sprigs of rosemary and a handful of chamomile flowers in a bowl. Add 10 fl oz (0.3 liters) freshly boiled water and leave to infuse until the water reaches room temperature. Strain the herbs out and add 3⅓ fl oz (100ml) lemon juice, then place the liquid in a bottle. Use as a final rinse after shampooing and conditioning your hair.

DRY SHAMPOO: If you have no time to shampoo your hair before going out, dust it with talcum powder or cornstarch and brush it out. Try this out first when you are not in a hurry to make sure that it works in the way you want.

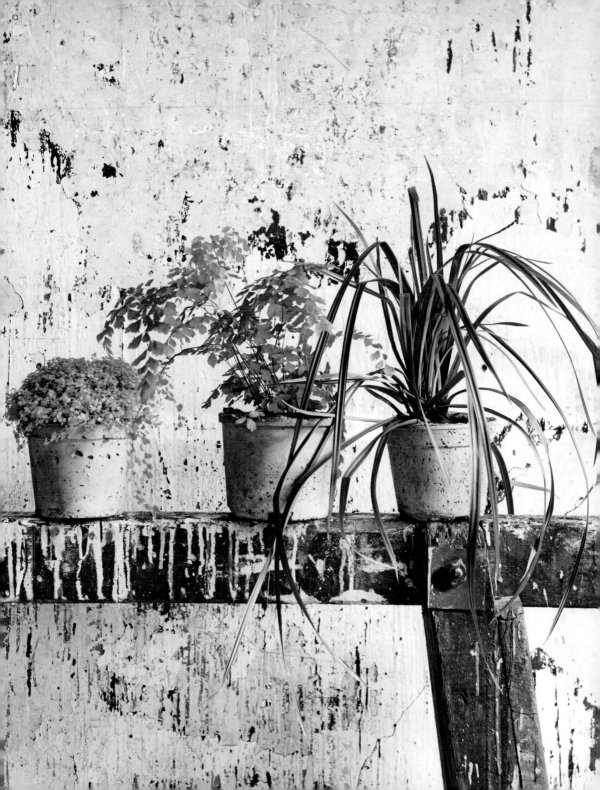

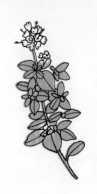

chapter 5

a healthy home and garden

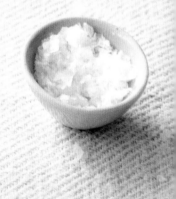

DIY all-purpose cleaner

Baking soda (bicarbonate of soda) is miraculous for tough stains, rust, ovens, tiles, tough grease, smelly fridges, and many other household problems—but don't use it on fine furniture or delicate fabrics.

1 teaspoon baking soda (bicarbonate of soda)

1 teaspoon liquid Castile soap

3 drops lemon essential oil or 1 teaspoon lemon juice

2 pints (1.2 liters) warm water

Put all the ingredients in a bowl and mix well, then transfer to a clean spray bottle and shake. For tougher-than-usual cleaning, add 1 cup (225 ml) white vinegar to the mix.

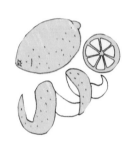

using homemade cleaners

When you start making your own cleaning products, it's important to bear the following points in mind.

BE CAREFUL: Use caution even with homey, organic ingredients, and avoid getting vinegar, lemon juice, borax, or any of your eco concoctions in your eyes.

USE IT OR LOSE IT!: Because they contain no preservatives, DIY cleaning mixes don't last very long, so use regularly for a clean green home!

WORTH THE WORK: Eco cleaning solutions take a bit more effort but are always worth it in the end. Not only are you saving money, but you are also making your home a healthier place for your family.

citrus floor cleanser

Commercial cleansers are chock full of chemicals and potential toxins, whereas simple herbal DIY cleaners are much healthier for you and your loved ones and always smell more natural. Who doesn't love the smell of lavender, citrus, and fresh mint?

juice of 2 limes
juice of 2 lemons
a handful of fresh mint
6 drops lavender essential oil

In a ceramic bowl, pour 2 cups (480ml) of hot water and half a cup (120ml) of lime and lemon juice, then add the fresh mint leaves and the lavender oil. Stir and let steep for a half hour, then strain out the leaves and compost them.

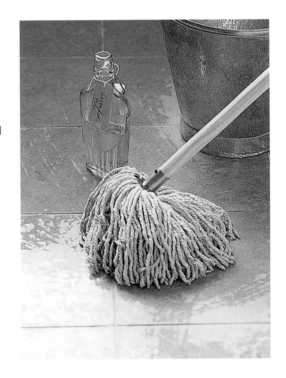

Take a clean bucket and fill it with two gallons of warm water, then pour in the essential oil mixture. Dip your mop into the bucket, wring it out, and clean the floor very thoroughly.

sage and cinnamon floor cleanser

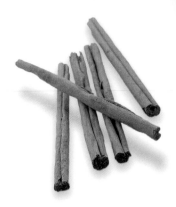

This is a wonderful floor wash for any purpose (although do leave out the lemon if your floor is delicate or made from antique wood).

1 cup (225 ml) hot water

3 sprigs mint

½ cup (110 ml) lemon juice (about 4 lemons)

8 drops lavender oil

3 sage leaves

3 cinnamon sticks

2 pints (1.2 liters) white vinegar

Pour the hot water into a large glass mixing bowl, and add the mint, lemon juice, lavender oil, sage leaves, and cinnamon sticks. Stir and let steep for a half hour.

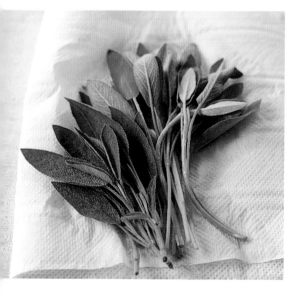

Fill a clean bucket with 2 gallons (7.5 liters) warm water and the white vinegar. Using a kitchen strainer (sieve), strain the herbal mix into the bucket and stir with a wooden spoon. Dip a brand-new mop into the bucket, wring it out, and clean the floor thoroughly.

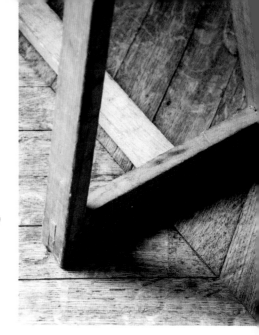

peppermint rodent repellent

Once a month, use peppermint oil in your floor cleaning water to ward off rodents. Keep a refillable spray bottle filled with a strong mixture of water and peppermint oil to spray around the outside of garbage cans, in the attic, and in the backs of closets.

good-for-wood eco floor cleaner

Your floors will look great and smell even better with this floor cleaner that's specially designed for wooden surfaces.

- 1 tablespoon white vinegar
- 1 tablespoon olive oil
- 5 drops lemon essential oil
- 2 pints (1.2 liters) warm water
- 1 drop lavender oil

Mix all the ingredients in a large glass bowl and pour into a clean spray bottle. Spray on the floor and wipe with a clean, damp mop. Follow by mopping with hot water. Allow the floor to dry a little and buff with a clean, dry cloth onto which you have sprinkled the lavender oil.

baking soda oven cleaner

Baking soda (bicarbonate of soda) can be used as an eco-friendly oven cleaner. When cleaning your oven—which is, after all, where you cook food for you and your family—it's better to skip chemicals, which leave an unhealthy residue.

water

vinegar (optional)

1 cup (140 g) baking soda (bicarbonate of soda)

Make a paste by adding a little water, or equal parts water and vinegar, to the baking soda. There will be a temporary foaming reaction so use a big bowl to avoid any mess and mix well. Use the paste to coat the inside of the oven and leave overnight.

In the morning, turn the oven on low heat for an hour, then leave to cool. Use a spray bottle of equal parts water and vinegar to soften the hardened paste, and use elbow grease to scrub it off. When you are baking that next batch of cookies for your loved ones, you can rest assured that no fumes will get into the yummy treat!

natural cleaning scrub

Baking soda (bicarbonate of soda) can also be used to make a general scrub. Mix ½ cup (140 g) baking soda with ¼ cup (60 ml) liquid Castile soap to make a paste the consistency of frosting. Scrub any surface that needs cleaning, then rinse with water. Do bear in mind that baking soda is slightly abrasive, so fragile fabrics and surfaces—including glass, mirrors, and antique or rare woods—may not fare well. Do a little test, then, if no problems arise, scrub to your heart's content.

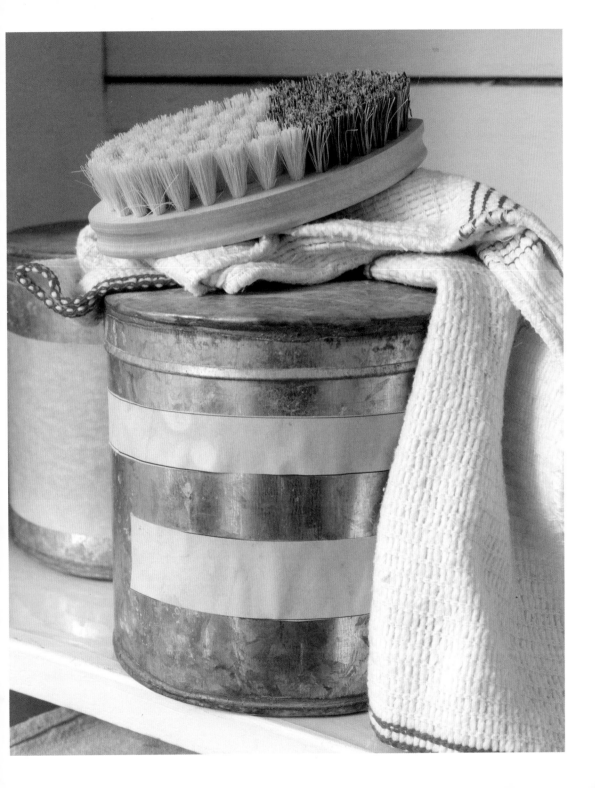

tea tree wipes

Instead of the toxic, chemical-laden wipes you can buy at the store, make your own to keep handy for unexpected spills and scheduled cleanings.

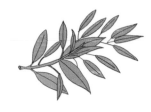

1 cup (225 ml) white vinegar
½ cup (110 ml) lemon juice
8 drops tea tree oil

Mix the white vinegar, lemon juice, and tea tree oil. Soak clean cloths or paper towels (kitchen towels) in the mixture and store in a screw-top jar or resealable bag for wipes that last up to a month.

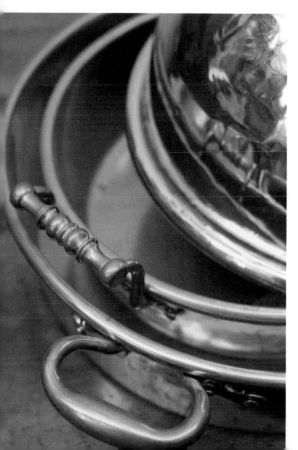

yogurt copper polish

Did you know your breakfast yogurt can be used to clean and polish copper pans, kitchen accessories, and basins?

Coat the copper with plain yogurt, leave it until it turns green (about 30 minutes), then wipe away with an old cloth. The copper will shine brilliantly.

coarse salt grease cleaner

Some people swear by scouring pots, pans, and cooking surfaces with salt.

It absorbs oil and grease, making it great for the stovetop, which can accumulate cooking splatters that are tough to remove. Sprinkle it on and scrub away with a damp sponge. You can also use salt with a lemon (see page 129).

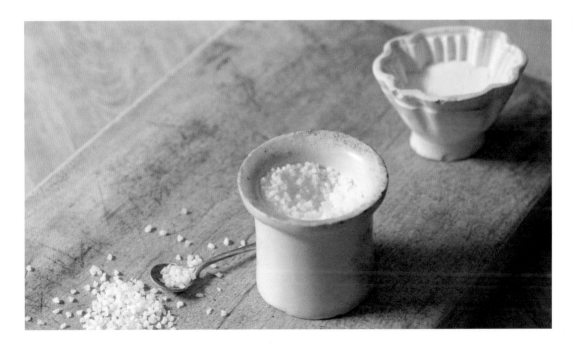

lemon power

For millennia, people have used lemon oil in washing water for clothes and linens, or cleaned their homes using hot water containing lemon leaves. The versatility of this beloved yellow fruit is fantastic. Instead of discarding lemon halves after you've used the juice for cooking or for making lemonade, save them to use around the home.

clean cheese graters

Cut a lemon in half and run it over the grater. The acid in the lemon will help to break down the fat in the cheese. If the food is really stuck on the grater, dip the lemon in table salt and the salt will act as a scrubber; combined with the lemon, it will remove most foods.

sanitize metal jewelry

The acid in lemon juice also removes tarnish. Use just ¼ cup (60 ml) freshly squeezed lemon juice to 1½ cups (335 ml) water. You can also dip your silver into a glass of fizzy lemon soda (lemonade) and it will come out sparkling. But don't use this combination on gold or pearls.

preserve meat and clean your cutting board

Lemon juice creates an acidic environment, and bacteria need an alkaline environment to survive, so adding lemon to meat, fresh produce, and even water inhibits bacterial growth. A handy antibacterial and natural way to clean your cutting board after cooking meat is to rub lemon juice on it and let it sit overnight, before rinsing it in the morning. The lemon juice will kill bacteria and leave your board smelling fresh.

naturally restore furniture and wood floors

Mix equal parts mayonnaise, olive oil, and lemon juice, and rub into wood furniture. This mix will add oil to the wood, and the lemon juice will cut through any build-up of polish. For floors, mix a little fresh lemon juice with olive oil.

brighten white tiles, sinks, and tubs

Mix fresh lemon juice with baking soda (bicarbonate of soda) and use to clean discolored ceramics before rinsing thoroughly.

prevent rice from sticking

Add 1 teaspoon lemon juice to the pot while the water is boiling to keep the grains from sticking together and to enhance the whiteness of your rice. Other citrus fruit has the same effect.

get rid of grease

Copper pots are cleaned quickly with half a lemon dipped in salt. Rub over a tarnished copper bottom pot and you'll see magic; the same combination works really well for removing grease from a stovetop and from stainless-steel pots and pans. For a real build-up of grease, this method is your go-to chemical-free solution.

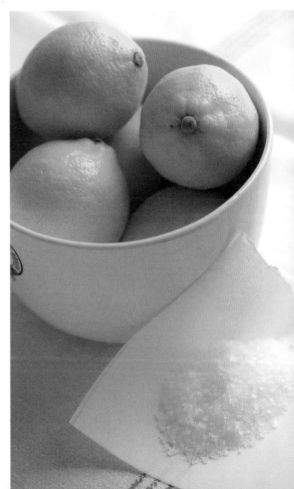

the scent of happiness

The minute you walk into someone's home, you can tell how happy a household it is. Much of that is determined by the smell. A space redolent of lilies or tea roses is obviously one whose occupants take care to make their home beautiful to the eye and the other senses.

2 drops neroli oil

4 drops bergamot oil

4 drops lavender oil

2 drops rosemary oil

2 pints (1.2 liters) distilled water

Combine the essential oils, then add the mixture to the distilled water in a spray bottle. Spray the air around the house.

removing odors

It's possible to get rid of unpleasant smells around the house without resorting to synthetic air fresheners.

COOKING: To rid the kitchen of cooking odors, simmer a solution of white distilled vinegar and water in a pan for 5 minutes.

GARBAGE CANS: Sprinkle baking soda into the bottom of garbage cans to remove unpleasant odors. After emptying the garbage, add some water and swill around the can. Pour it out and leave to dry, then add more baking soda for next time.

DRAINS: To deodorize drains, pour a cup of white distilled vinegar down the drain and leave for half an hour, then flush through with running cold water. A mixture of vinegar and baking soda will do the job even more thoroughly. Pour two tablespoons of baking soda down the sink hole followed by half a cup of vinegar, leave to bubble for 20 minutes, then flush through by running the cold faucet (tap) for a minute.

CARPETS: Sprinkle baking soda (bicarbonate of soda) over carpets to deodorize them. Leave for an hour, then vacuum.

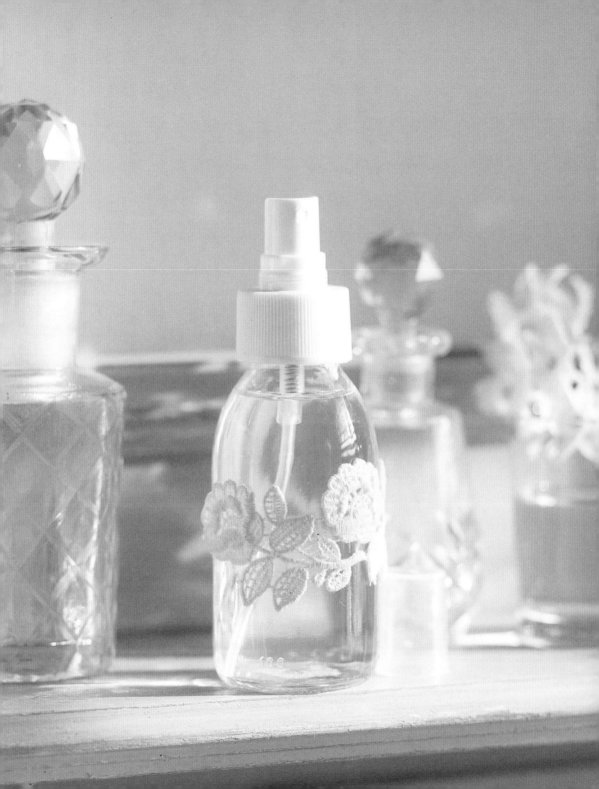

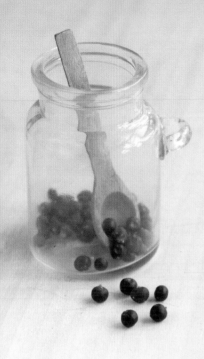

power potpourri

Simmer this mixture in a pot of water on your stove whenever you feel the need to infuse your space with positive energy.

¼ cup (5 g) dried rosemary

4 dried bay laurel leaves

⅛ cup (5 g) dried sage

1 teaspoon dried juniper berries

Mix the herbs together by hand, then add them to the slowly simmering water and breathe in the newly charged air.

purifying plants

Did you know that houseplants can improve the air we breathe? They purify the air by producing oxygen and absorbing contaminants, like formaldehyde and benzene, which are commonly off-gassed by furniture and mattresses. Try keeping bamboo, weeping fig, rubber tree, spider plant, peace lily, or snake plant.

Houseplants need their leaves dusted and you can do this with a banana peel. The dust clings to the peel and the leaves are nourished by it.

happy home spray

This blend smells wonderful, almost like you're walking through an orchard in full bloom. The aroma is fresh, fortifying, fruity, and floral. Neroli is excellent for calm and reducing anxiety, lemon refreshes and uplifts, while tangerine sends sadness away, and quickly. Spritz this happy home spray in shared space, such as the living room, and in your bedroom for optimal rest and restoration. You can also very lightly spritz it on linens and towels.

2 fl oz (60 ml) distilled water

6 drops neroli essential oil

6 drops lemon essential oil

6 drops tangerine essential oil

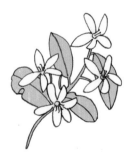

Fill a 2-fl oz (60-ml) spray bottle with the distilled water, leaving room at the top for the oils. Add in the essential oils and then seal the lid tightly. Shake vigorously and it's ready for use.

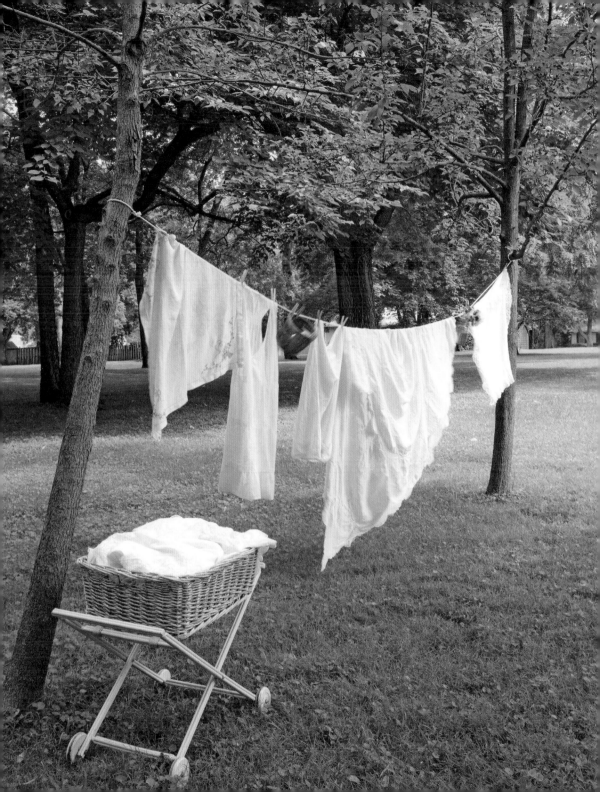

eco laundry detergent

Want to get away from the chemicals, foaming agents, and synthetic fragrances found in most laundry detergents? This one will work beautifully in cold or warm cycles.

bar of pure soap (ideally frozen)

1 cup (140 g) borax

1 cup (140 g) washing soda

lemon juice (optional)

Use a box grater to grate the soap bar into a powder (it is easiest if you freeze the soap first). Mix the powder with the borax, washing soda, and a few drops of lemon juice, if using. Use 1 or 2 tablespoons of your detergent per load.

secrets to stain removal

Try these ingenious solutions to avoid permanent unsightly marks on your clothes and linens.

TABLE SALT: If you spill coffee or red wine on your couch, carpet, or tablecloth, pour plain table salt into the spill immediately and it will soak it right up. The salt turning purple-blue as it soaks up red wine is truly spellbinding! Vacuum it up and the stain will be gone.

BAKING SODA: Soak stained clothes, towels, and bed linens in cold water with baking soda (bicarbonate of soda) or white vinegar, and wash in cold water only to avoid "setting" the stain.

BORAX: There is no need to use bleach for white fabrics in your laundry: Use 1 cup (140 g) borax instead. Alternatively, throw discolored white cotton socks, towels, or shirts in a stockpot with water and a few used lemons and simmer for a little while to lighten. (Only do this with pure cotton fabrics, and do not attempt this method with anything containing elastic.) If you hang them outside to dry, the combination of sun and your low-cost lemon whitener will refresh them until they are practically gleaming!

compost tea

Compost tea is a marvelous way to feed your plants and give them extra nutrients in a wholly natural way that is free of chemicals.

2 cups (400 g) fresh, homemade compost from your compost bin, pile, or garden center

1 gallon (3.75 liters) clean, filtered water

Put the compost and water in a large bucket and place out of direct heat or cold—a shed or a garage will do nicely. Let your compost tea "brew" for a week and give it a stir every other day. When the time is up, strain out the dirt and pour the liquid into your watering can—the perfect garden teapot—to serve up some serious nutrients to your plants.

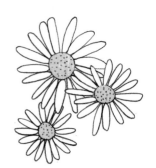

lemon in the garden

Not only is lemon wonderfully helpful in your house (see pages 128–129), but it also has uses outdoors, too.

deter pests

Lemon rinds placed around the border of your herb and flower garden will keep away pests, ranging from insects to pets and animals.

kill weeds

Forget chemical weedkillers, which can be just as bad for you as they are for the planet. Control weeds with a lemon and white vinegar mixture, which is four parts lemon juice to one part white vinegar. Pour into a spray bottle, shake well, and head out into the garden, taking care to spray only the weeds. They will shrivel and die, making them easy to pull out and compost.

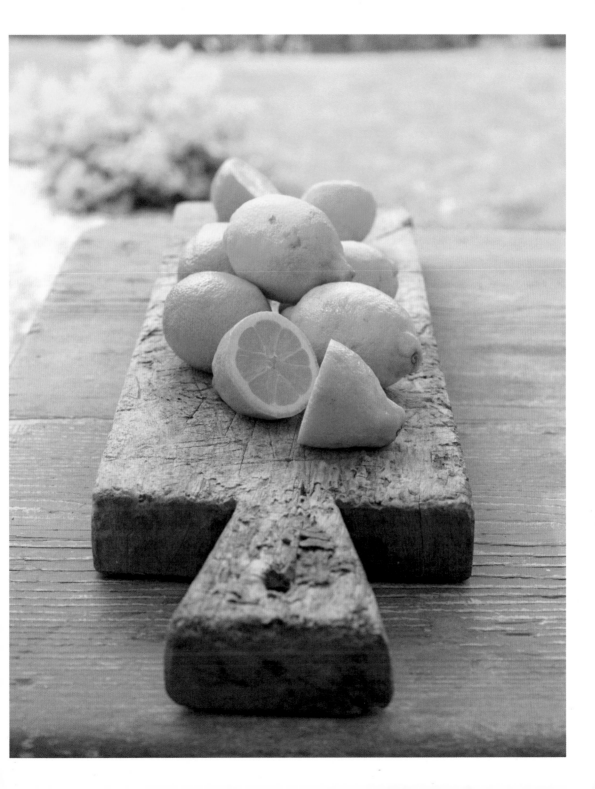

herbal plant spray

To keep your herbs, vegetables, and fruits free from insects and snails, use this spray on them.

¾ oz (20 g) chili

10 red peppercorns

3 whole wild garlic (or 5 garlic cloves if you cannot find wild)

3 citronella leaves

¾ fl oz (20 g) mild fluid soap (preferably odorless)

Add 3¾ fl oz (100ml) water and the herbs to a blender and blend until completely smooth. Pour into a spray bottle. Add soap and fill up with water. Spray your garden when there is no direct sunlight.

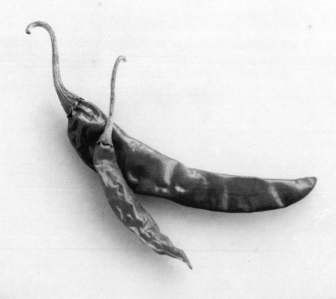

flea-repellent pet pillow

Discourage fleas with this herbal mix.

2 oz (50 g) dried pennyroyal

¾ oz (20 g) dried thyme

¾ oz (20 g) dried wormwood

¾ oz (20 g) dried catnip

Mix together all the ingredients. If your dog or cat has a special bed, you can open a seam and sprinkle the herbs inside to create a flea-repellant pet bed. If you like to cover your pet with a fleece or they like to lay on one, rub some of the herbal mixture into the fleece.

insect repellent for dogs

To keep tiny, irritating insects away from your dog, add a few drops of geranium essential oil to the last rinse during a bath, or rub the oil into his or her neck.

herbal insect repellent

This works especially well to ward off mosquitoes in summer when you have the windows open at night.

5 citronella leaves

5 basil leaves

5 mint leaves

5 cloves

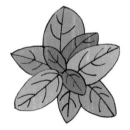

Place the herbs in the middle of a square of organza. Bring up the corners and tie with a ribbon to make a little round parcel. Place in windows, on outdoors tables, or in closets.

resources

herbs, spices, and adaptogens

ABC.HERBALGRAM.ORG
The journal of the American Botanical Council includes a database of herbs and their uses.

BOTANICAL.COM
Great online herbal encyclopedia.

MOUNTAINROSEHERBS.COM
U.S. supplier of organic herbs (including ethically wild-harvested and Kosher certified botanical products), spices, loose-leaf teas, essential oils, and herbal extracts.

BANYANBOTANICALS.COM
Another U.S. option for herbs and spices, including triphala (as well as essential oils). Its products are organic.

SCARLETSAGE.COM
San Francisco-based supplier of dried herbs, essential oils, floral waters, and books.

SUNPOTION.COM
International supplier of herbs and adaptogens, including triphala.

DANDELIONBOTANICAL.COM
U.S. natural apothecary supplying certified organic herbs, spices, and botanicals.

MADDOCKSFARMORGANICS.CO.UK
Huge variety of organic edible flowers grown in Devon, England, UK.

You can also source many organic herbs in bulk from Amazon, Whole Foods, or your local boutique natural medicine shops.

essential oils and bath salts

WWW.AROMAWEB.COM/ARTICLES/SAFETY.ASP
Advice on using essential oils safely.

MAPI.COM AND MAHARISHI.CO.UK
Maharishi Ayurveda is hosts high-quality massage oils and Ayurvedic herbs (such as triphala) and lifestyle supplements.

YOUNGLIVING.COM/EN_US AND YOUNGLIVING.COM/EN_GB
Young Living carries an array of essential oils, household cleaning solutions, supplements, and body-care and baby products.

SEASALT.COM
SaltWorks carries organic Epsom salts in bulk. If you are planning on taking plenty of baths, you could purchase the 50 lb (22.6 kg) bag. You can also find Epsom salts at your local pharmacy and health food store.

index

adaptogens 14–15, 107
  adaptogenic beauty milk 99
allspice 13
  and oregano healing bath 32
almond 16
  and grapefruit joy lotion 112
aloe vera 36, 60
anxiety 71, 75, 83, 87
apple cider vinegar 49, 96
  hair conditioner 116
apple mint and meadowsweet
    calmer 80

baking soda 77, 120, 129, 130,
    135
  oven cleaner 124
  shampoo 116
balm 11
  bay leaf balm to de-stress 82
  mood-boosting blends 109
  neroli and vanilla calming
    balm 108
  raspberry lip balm 110
basil 9, 61, 71
baths 73, 74, 77
  detox 107
  moisturizing coconut 114
  oregano and allspice
    healing 32
  relaxing chamomile 106
  rose milk 106
  sprinkle for peace 72
bay 9
  leaf balm to de-stress 82
bergamot 9, 71, 75
birch
  ginger and wisteria detoxer 52
  sap 53
blackberry 16
  tonic for tummy aches and
    cramps 25
blood pressure 49, 56
blueberry 16
borax, stain remover 135
breathe easy salt 20

calm emotion potion 68
cardamom 13, 52, 57
carrier oil 12
carrot, ginger soup 23
catnip 11
  tea 27
celery 17
  juice elixir 56
cinnamon 13, 52
  and sage floor cleanser 122
chamomile 10, 71, 79
  brightening fair hair 117
  face mask 90
  and lavender tranquility
    tonic 78
  relaxing bath 107
  strengthening hair rinse 117
cholesterol 49
citrus floor cleanser 121
citrus-rose hydrosol 97
clove 14
  and elderberry syrup 43
coconut, moisturizing bath 114
colds 20, 23, 25, 33, 41, 42
comfrey and lavender salve 35
compost tea 136
coughs 20, 21, 25, 33
  teas 22
cucumber 17
  lotion 36
cumin 13, 55

dandelion 50
  sassafras and ginger detox 51
detox 50, 51, 52, 54, 55. 56, 61
  bath 106
digestion 26–27, 42, 55, 56, 57,
    58, 60
digestive rose tea 57
DIY all-purpose cleaner 120

echinacea root tea 41
eco laundry detergent 135
elderberry
  and clove syrup 43

flu buster 42
energy 49
essential oils 64, 71
  blends 65, 66, 68, 69, 72, 75

fennel 10, 26, 55, 57
  ginger and lemon thyme
    reviver 54
fever 23, 25
  tea 24
flea-repellent pet pillow 139
flower essences 85–87
foot, mint miracle therapy 113

gardener's tea for aching joints
    30
ginger 14, 57
  birch and wisteria detoxer
    52
  and carrot soup 23
  dandelion and sassafras
    detox 51
  fennel and lemon thyme
    reviver 54
  syrup 43
good-for-wood eco floor
    cleaner 123
gout 28
grapefruit and almond joy
    lotion 112
gripe water 27

haircare, homemade 116
happy home spray 133
hay fever 44
headache 33, 77
healing aloe 60
herbal plant spray 138
herbs 8–12
honey 21
  and lavender mocktail 44–45
  thyme 31
hops 47
horsetail hair tonic 117

immune system boosting 40, 41, 42
insect repellent 72
    for dogs 139
    herbal 139

jasmine 10, 71
joint pain 24, 30, 35

kitchari, modern reset 58

laundry
    eco detergent 135
    stain removal 135
    thyme 133
lavender 8, 45, 70, 71, 75, 79
    and chamomile tranquility
        tonic 78
    and comfrey salve 35
    and honey mocktail 44–45
    and lemon lift blend 68
    infusion 33
    to help headaches 33
    tea 33
    tincture 34
lemon 17, 133, 135
    and lavender lift blend 68
    in the garden 136
    power 128–9
    and water digestion aid 56–7
lemon balm 12, 71
lemon thyme, fennel and ginger
        reviver 54
licorice 16, 50
lips
    nourishing lip gloss 109
    raspberry lip balm 110
lotions
    cucumber 36
    pulse-point 70
    grapefruit and almond joy 112

magnesium 15, 28, 73, 107
masks
    chamomile face mask 90
    blossoming beauty mask 93
    moringa mermaid mask 91
    sandalwood shakti mask 92
massage, blissful bars 114
    oil 68, 69, 72

meadowsweet 81
    and apple mint calmer 80
    syrup 81
mint miracle foot therapy 113
modern kitchari reset 58
moringa 15
    mermaid mask 91
    morning matcha tonic 95
muscular pain 30, 32, 35, 54, 83

natural remedy blends 66
neroli 133
    and vanilla calming balm 108
nettle 16
    scalp tonic 117
nutmeg 13, 92
    milk 27

odors, removing 130
oils
    ageless skin potion 100
    beautifying 99
    carrier 12
    essential 64
    glowing goddess face 94
    self-massage 102
ointment 11
orange and spice blend 72
oregano 8
    and allspice healing bath 32
oxymel tonic 21

parsley seed hair tonic 117
patchouli 9, 71
peppermint 8
    oil for muscular pain 32
    rodent repellent 123
plants, purifying 132
    compost tea 136
    grow your own aloe 60
    herbal spray 138
power potpourri 132
pulse-point lotion 70

quiet mind tea 79

raspberry lip balm 110
red clover 10
    lemonade 28

relaxation massage oil blend 69
restorative infusion for energy 49
revitalizing herb tea 78
rose 71, 98
    citrus-rose hydrosol 97
    digestive tea 57
    milk bath 106
    renewal spray 96
rose hip tea 40
rosemary 8, 75
    adding shine to dark hair 117
    strengthening hair rinse 117

saffron and lemon elixir 100
sage 8
    and cinnamon floor cleanser
        122
    lotion 36
Saint-John's-wort 36
salt 129, 135
    breathe easy 20
    coarse salt grease cleaner 127
    dead sea 105
    scrub to relax and aid sleep 73
salve 11, 31
    comfrey and lavender cure-all
        35
sandalwood shakti mask 92
sassafras, dandelion and ginger
        detox 51
scent of happiness, the 130
scrubs
    body purification salt 105
    salt scrub to relax and aid
        sleep 73
    yummy spa 104
self-massage 102–3
sensual soak 77
skin-nourishing body whip 113
skin problems 34, 35, 36
skullcap tincture for comfort and
        calm 83
sleep problems 33, 47, 73
    milk 46
    tea 46
soothing stomach tea 24
spices 13–14
stain removal secrets 135
sterilizing 17

stress relief 68, 79, 82
stomach problems 24, 25, 26–27, 30, 33, 34, 54

teas
  beauty ambrosia tea 98
  catnip 27
  cough 22
  digestive rose 57
  echinacea root 41
  fever 24
  gardener's tea for aching joints 30
  gentle detox 55
  green 61
  lavender 33
  quiet mind 79
  restorative infusion for energy 49
  revitalizing herb 78
  rose hip 40
  sleep 46
  soothing stomach 24

vitali-tea 50
vitamin C 40
weight-loss 61
tea tree wipes 126
thyme 12
  laundry 133
  tincture 31
tincture
  lavender 34
  skullcap, for comfort and calm 83
  thyme 31
tonics
  blackberry 25
  lavender and chamomile tranquility 78
  moringa morning matcha 95
  oxymel 21
triphala 26

valerian 12, 47, 71, 79
vanilla 70
  and neroli calming balm 108

vinegar 17
  apple cider 49
  blackberry 25
  distilled 127, 130
  malt vinegar hair tonic 117
vitali-tea 50
vitamin C tea 40

walking 26
water
  gripe 27
  and lemon digestion aid 56–57
waters of wellness 74
weight-loss tea 61
wounds 30, 34, 35

ylang ylang 71, 75, 114
yogurt copper polish 126

credits

photography credits

PHOTOGRAPHY © CICO BOOKS/RYLAND PETERS AND SMALL
Caroline Arber: pp. 22, 31, 47, 117, 120; Hans Blomquist: p. 123; Martin Brigdale: pp. 21, 95; Peter Cassidy: pp. 27, 30, 32, 33, 56, 57, 63, 82, 86, 116, 122; Helen Cathcart: p. 23; Stephen Conroy: pp. 15, 59, 98, 101; Belle Daughtry: pp. 1, 2, 4–5, 6, 9, 11, 12, 41, 48, 62, 65, 67, 69, 75, 76, 87, 105; Tara Fisher: p. 72; Michelle Garrett: p. 45; Richard Jung: p. 26; Mowie Kay: pp. 104, 111; Kim Lightbody: pp. 18, 24, 29, 34, 53, 54, 80, 84; William Lingwood: p. 122; Mark Lohman: p. 134; Peter Moore: p. 81; Gloria Nicol: pp. 42, 129; Steve Painter: pp. 25, 61; William Reavell: pp. 90, 132; Claire Richardson: pp. 73, 127; Lucinda Symons: pp. 17, 35, 37, 125, 126, 137; Debi Treloar: pp. 60 (Nicky Philips' apartment in London), 106;

Ian Wallace: pp. 38, 99; Stuart West: pp. 88, 94, 96, 115, 131; Clare Winfield: pp. 39, 119; Kate Whitaker: pp. 19, 55, 89, 112, 138; Rachel Whiting: p. 118; Polly Wreford: p. 102; Penny Wincer: p. 20.

PHOTOGRAPHY FROM SHUTTERSTOCK
p. 83 © Mariola Anna S; p. 91 © Lukas Gojda; p. 92 © drebha; p. 93 © artcasta; p. 97 © July Prokopiv.

author credits